Shoulder Down

TODD PAYETTE

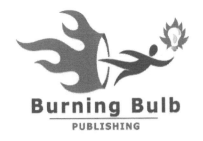

Burning Bulb
PUBLISHING

Shoulder Down
By **Todd Payette**

Burning Bulb Publishing
P.O. Box 4721
Bridgeport, WV 26330-4721
United States of America
www.BurningBulbPublishing.com

Cover photos by Marcin and Dawid Witukiewicz of Bombelkie Photography.

First Edition.

Paperback Edition ISBN: 978-1-948278-44-7

"For my mother, Lucille.
The strongest person I've ever known."

ACKNOWLEDGEMENTS

A special thank you to those of you that have always had my back. No man succeeds alone.

My sister Linda. I look up to you in so many ways. So tough, smart, funny. You have always rooted for me. I still think you could probably kick my ass if needed!

My closest friends, Rob Kliewer and Trevor King. Thank you for putting up with all my crap through the years! The laughter kept me sane.

Syd Korsynsky and Ken Kelsh. My basketball coaches from Elmwood High. Shoulder down is a life lesson that has served me well.

Aubrey Daniels. You took a chance on me when nobody else would. Thank you.

Ralph Eannace. Like my big brother. Always there to listen and give advice and support. Always in my corner. You are an amazing man.

Si Sweeney. What can I say about you? You inspire me to be the best version of myself. You are a blessing in my life.

Val and Jim Charles along with Eddy Ellwood. You gave me a shot at living my dream. Competing at the NABBA Mr. Universe. The word that best describes you all...CLASS!!!

Richard Politano. Friend, iron brother and world class coach. Your knowledge and honesty drives me to be my best. I'm in your debt.

Jeni Briscoe. World class bodybuilder, trainer and friend. As solid as they come. You gave me a great opportunity that I value every day!!!

Dian Wiebe. The kindest heart I know. Words can't express my feelings. So, I try to show you every day. Thank you for walking beside me. Also for tolerating my humour. You have my heart.

Mike Torchia. Not only a bodybuilding legend but a true brother in iron. You are an inspiration. It was you who encouraged me to write this book. Thank you for your help and always providing sound advice!

To those that I may have missed. All the bodybuilders, Elmwood people, all of you that have followed my bizarre and crazy story. Thank you.

Gary Lee Vincent. My partner in this crazy venture. Thank you for believing, and all your hard work. This would not have been possible without your guidance and expertise!

CHAPTER 1

"I bet it ain't cookie dough."

Having a gun pointed at your head is generally a good sign that you are about to have a very bad day.

This particular day was going to be one of those days. When I saw the flashing lights, heard the sirens, I did as anyone would do. I pulled over to the right and stopped my car. I remember thinking, "holy shit, that's a lot of cops. A few seconds later, I have a handgun pointed at my temple while another officer screams at me to get out of my car! The pistol is at my right temple, passenger side. The shouting is from my left. It's a warm night and my windows were all down.

"GET THE FUCK OUT OF THE CAR NOW!!!" I was in shock. WHAT WAS GOING ON? I reached down to unfasten my seat belt. CRACK!!! The punch stunned me. Not that I hadn't been punched in my life. It was a very familiar feeling. More than anything, at that moment, I was mad. I turn to my left, standing there is a cop, in his best *I'm a badass undercover cop wear*. A ginger, covered in tats, about 6 feet tall, 160 lbs, soaking wet. He saw his opportunity for a free shot, and he took it. At 6 feet tall, 220 lbs of muscle, I barely felt it. Still, I was pissed.

"REALLY?!!" I shouted at him. "I have to undo the seat belt to get out!" They kept shouting at me. I followed their instructions to the letter, with zero resistance on my part. As far as I could tell, three of them jumped on me, forcing me to the ground, shredding my favorite old gym tank top off in the process.

"Damn," I thought. "Love that shirt." Funny what you think about in a situation like this. Everything seemed to slow down.

More yelling. One cop shouts, "Why were you in Calgary?"

They throw me against the back of a cruiser and place two sets of handcuffs on me and proceed to put me in the back of the cruiser.

I remember thinking, "Two sets of handcuffs!? Do they think I'm going to turn green?

5

I was tired. I had driven non-stop from Calgary and was a block from getting home. I wanted to see my dogs, my girlfriend, Denise. Add to that, I was preparing to compete in the Provincial Bodybuilding Championships in a week. The depletion you put your body through is exhausting. Low or no carbs make it tough to focus and drains the body's physical energy. "What the hell is this about?" was the thought that kept running through my head.

One of the officers slid into the front seat of the cruiser. He asked one question" What is in the package?"

UGH! THE PACKAGE!!! I didn't even think of that. I replied, "I have NO idea!" In hindsight, his reply was pretty damn funny. "Well, I bet it ain't cookie dough!"

He was right; it was NOT cookie dough!

CHAPTER 2

"The Milkman and Jack LaLanne."

My father was literally the milkman. He delivered milk for Silverwood Dairies. To this day, I remember the truck, the smell of the place, and how freezing cold the freezers were. The few times he brought me to work were amazing. He would let me wear his hat, which smelled of Brylcreem. It was hard not to feel important! He was the MILKMAN! For a 5-year-old boy, it was very impressive; the big truck, the uniform. He was like Superman to me!

His name was Andre. Everyone called him Andy. A wiry man with slick dark hair and sharp features, he resembled Hank Williams. From all accounts, he was well-liked by everyone. He bowled in a league with my Mother (more about her later). He smoked as most everyone did in those days. He grew up in a small town in Manitoba, Miami, I believe. Or close to there. French-speaking and very hard drinking family, the Payette's were and still are!

He was prone to seizures, as he had epilepsy. I found this out as an adult. There was much I was to learn later about the man I simply knew as "Dad."

Like many little boys, I wanted to be just like him. He bowled, so I loved bowling (still do). He loved chicken wings, so of course, it was my favorite! When he got ready for work in the morning, I would get ready along with him, and in my imagination, I was going with him to ride in the big dairy truck. He would go out back to the garage and would always circle around to the front of the house so I could watch him drive off. I would be on my little trike, pretending that I, too, was off to work at the dairy. When he got home at the end of the day, it was like God himself had walked in. Such was my admiration for him. He would give me his hat more often than not after I greeted him with a hug. My older sister, by two years, Linda, never welcomed him home. It was odd, they did not seem close, and she preferred her own company, staying in her room when not called upon to eat dinner or some chore or another.

We ate as a family. My Mother always had a decent meal for us all—standard fare, meat, a veggie, and almost always potatoes. Unless mashed, I absolutely detested them. The rule was you ate everything on your plate and stayed at the table until this was done. Linda ALWAYS finished everything, which I hated her for. Damn, she even ate the green beans! Our younger sister, Tina, was a baby, and I was the dreaded "picky eater"! I could eat almost any type of meat, which would serve me well later. However, as a child, it was hard for me to choke down veggies or anything else! I spent many an evening slowly getting through dinner while everyone else was in the living room watching TV. Sometimes, I would try and hide my food in the garbage, would get busted, and a beating followed—all in all, a good trade-off. I could take the beating. I mean, it was a spanking. By today's standards, that would be abuse. Laughable!

HOCKEY NIGHT IN CANADA! I still remember the theme music! If it was on, Dad was watching it. I loved watching the little black puck whiz along the ice with amazing speed. The impossibly large-shouldered players (I didn't realize they wore padding), and the best part was watching with Dad.

He favored me. I was his son, his boy. Linda largely ignored him, and I think he did the same to her. Tina would cry if Mom left the room; she had colic and seemed to be crying almost all the time. She was a baby. I got the attention from Dad, which suited me just fine. Watching hockey with him, I had a job. I got him his beer. It was, to me, a very important job. I went to the fridge, got a bottle, opened it, took a sip, and brought it to him. I definitely would be feeling it by bedtime. I was a man, after all, like Dad. Of course, I would drink some. He laughed. He knew. He didn't care. His whole family drank and drank hard. It was really a rite of passage. In his mind, he pictured us drinking together one day, of that I am quite sure. Just as he drank with his Dad, and my uncles. He was a happy drunk. He was an alcoholic.

My Dad was not afraid of hard work, however. I remember him coming home after job number two: delivering pizza for Pizza Place. One of the first pizza chains in Winnipeg, they had a fleet of VW Beetles for their delivery drivers. Some nights he would bring pizza home. Mom would wake us up for a late-night pizza snack. It was amazing! The pepperoni was his and, of course, my favorite. I would eat until I fell asleep. I never had problems eating pizza. He would sometimes carry Linda and me to bed. These were my happiest times.

Of course, when your father is an alcoholic, things were not all rainbows and sunshine. When we lived in an apartment, Linda and I shared a room. I remember us looking at each other as our parents had awful fights. Both of us were terrified of the yelling. I would ask her to make it stop, and she would motion for me to be quiet as we hid in our beds. It was scary. Sometimes things would get smashed. I hated it, hated the feeling of fear. The next day, nothing would be said, and life would carry on.

We eventually moved out of the apartment to a duplex in Elmwood, a tough, blue-collar neighborhood in Winnipeg. We were just across the river from the much tougher North End and on a busy street. We had a yard! With swings and a sandbox to our delight. My Dad had a garage for his car, which made him very happy. We had our own rooms, and it was all very impressive to me.

It seemed things were good for our little family.

Sometimes Dad didn't come home. I suppose many of the fights my parents had were about him vanishing for a couple of days.

We were not allowed in our parent's room, especially early in the morning. I had a pretty good system for finding out if he had come home. I went to the garage. If the car was there, he was home, life was good. My little world made sense. Sometimes he came home in the wee hours of the night. I always woke up when this happened. I never was a good sleeper and have sleep issues to this day. We had a ritual for when he staggered in. I would greet him and tell him I was hungry. I always had two choices: milk and cookies or cereal. He would fix it up for me and sit with me until I was done. Then he would bring me back to bed and stumble off to his room with my Mom. He always did this. Every time, without fail, if I woke up. Sometimes we would talk a little as I ate. Sometimes not. Just him and I. It was always apparent to me that he was at least a little drunk and sometimes, a lot drunk. That did not matter to me. It didn't scare me. It was our time together without my Mom, and better yet, without my crying baby sister and without Linda, who I saw as the "perfect" child that never got into trouble. Just father and son.

***

9

1974. It was a beautiful warm sunny Sunday morning. I was the only one awake, and Linda was at church with a school friend. After a bit of cereal and some morning television, it was time for me to check the garage to see if Dad was home. If he had come home in the night, I had slept through it as there had been no cereal or milk ritual.

Our garage was a two-car garage with lots of room and had that familiar smell of oil and gas as many garages do. As I approached the door, I noticed a sound coming from within, it was our car, and it was running. The image took me by surprise. There was Dad, slumped slightly to the left in our big blue Pontiac, door closed, window open, engine running. I remember an awful feeling as I called out weakly to him, "Dad?"

No response.

I opened the car door and climbed on his lap. Something was wrong. I called out to him again, louder, "DADDY!?"

Nothing.

I started to feel ill from the fumes, and something told me to turn off the car. I suppose watching every move my father made served me well as I knew exactly how to do it. I was feeling not so good from the exhaust, and I shudder to think what could have happened had I not turned it off. I was in there for at least 15 minutes, if not more, and it felt wrong to leave him. I tried shaking him, calling to him, hugging him. I turned on the radio loudly. I didn't want to leave him. After several minutes and with great effort, I knew I had to get help. I had to tell Mom.

I ran into the house full speed and burst into my parent's bedroom. I was shaking and could barely get the words out, "Mommy, Daddy is in the car, he's asleep, and he won't wake up!"

Never before or since had I seen my Mother move so fast. It didn't seem to make any sense to me, and I didn't even know she could run! Everything that happened immediately after that was a blur of sirens, fire trucks, and an ambulance. Curious folks from our street rubbernecked to see what was going on, and I was kept away from the garage.

To this day, I feel quite badly for the firefighter who came to speak to me. He gently put his hand on my shoulder and quietly said to me, "Son, I am very sorry, your father has died." The pain I felt in my stomach was immediate and intense. There was nothing I could say. I simply ran to my room and curled up on my bed, and howled. The pain would not stop; I was screaming.

After a few minutes, my Mom sat on the edge of my bed and began speaking to me. It was the first time in my memories that I remember her really talking to me. Before that moment, even though we spent every day together, my attention was devoted to my Dad. Unfair to her. Children are selfish wee buggers. She was there to feed me, give me a hard time when I needed it, teach me everything I needed to know. She parented 80% to my father's 20%, but to me, he was the hero.

"Todd, don't cry. It's going to be ok. You have to be the man now. It will be ok. Please don't cry." Understandably, I think she was at a loss. She was trying to console a little boy who had just found his father dead. All the while dealing with the fact that her husband was now gone, she had three kids under the age of nine, and now what the hell was she going to do?! The fact that she held it together at all is an excellent example of intestinal fortitude that I have not seen many times in my life. She was the hero.

After the situation had died down and with me in a state of shock, I asked my Mom if I could go down the street to my friend Daphne's house. She said yes. I found Daphne in the backyard of her house. She was coloring. I asked if I could watch. She said yes. I sat down next to her. The sun was warm on my shoulders. That perfect sort of warm. Not too hot, not enough to make you sweat. I watched her color and then watched some of her crayons melting slowly on the sidewalk.

The next day, I went to school. Nothing was said about anything. My Mom got me dressed, and off I went, business as usual. Things were different then. No one thought that perhaps crawling around your dead father's lap could leave a lasting and perhaps negative impression. If they thought it, nothing was said about it. They didn't let me go to the funeral either. So surreal. No goodbye. One day he was there, then poof! Gone.

My last memory of him was him in the garage. That memory is as clear as if it happened yesterday. To this day, I do not much like being in anyone's garage. Smell is a very strong trigger for memories. All garages seem to have that same smell, well, especially older ones. Newer houses not so much as no one works on their own cars anymore.

It was recess time at school not long after his death that it really hit me. I was playing by myself, and I started thinking of Dad. All of a sudden, it hit me like a punch to the gut, the finality of it all. I would never see my Dad again. I could not stop crying. The pain in my stomach was back. They sent me home. My Mom let me curl up in my bed, and I stayed there until the middle of the night. I woke up. An idea came to me. I went to the kitchen and made myself a bowl of cereal. In my little brain (remember, at this age, we believe in Santa and the Easter bunny), I surmised that if I made the cereal, he would come back. I sat there, milk and cereal all over the place, eating and sobbing and hoping it would work. Of course, it didn't. To this day, if I wake up in the middle of the night, nine out of ten times, I will eat cereal or cookies to go back to sleep.

Not sure how long after his death that I was introduced to the world of exercise. My best guess is that it was a few weeks at most. I was up early, making forts out of the sofa cushions with the television on in the background. Suddenly, I heard an energetic voice from the TV exclaiming, "Through exercise, you can live a long and healthy life!"

A long and healthy life? This grabbed my attention immediately as a dark fear of death had started plaguing me since the "incident" involving the garage. I watched as a small muscular man started performing various calisthenics all while talking; not out of breath, it looked effortless! Beautiful even. His movements were perfect. He had this tiny waist, broad shoulders, a shock of thick hair, and muscular arms. The influence was immediate, and it was profound. He exuded health and strength! He was nothing like my Dad, who, although wiry, was not the picture of vitality.

I wanted that strength! I wanted to live! I didn't want to die! This is how it began. The little muscular man on TV? Jack LaLanne. Six years old, push-ups, sit ups, jumping jacks as Jack encouraged me.

From that moment on, the focus of my life had totally changed. It would now be about being the fastest, the strongest, and a need to be different than anyone else.

I was not going to die. I was NOT going to be weak. It became extremely important that I was different than everyone else. I would listen to Jack.

CHAPTER 3

"I am not normal."

After the passing of my Dad, and my newfound mission of being stronger, healthier, and faster than everyone on the planet (remember, at five years old we have no understanding of the scale of our world and population), my young mind decided and felt that I was different than everyone else. Not better by any stretch, just different.

Perhaps it's normal for any child after experiencing a traumatic event to feel "different." For myself, the best way to explain it was that innocence was lost. My humour became somewhat morbid for a little kid, and some things affected me way more than others.

For example, after witnessing a dog being hit by a car in front of my house, I felt physically ill and could not leave my room until the next day. By contrast, we had neighbors that lived below us in our duplex. They had two children, Kim and Tim. Kim was one year younger than me and was my friend. She had a brain tumour. Due to her treatments, she lost all her hair and wore wigs to school. I was very protective of her. Her family moved away about a year or so after my Dad's death. After school one day, my mother took me aside and said, "I have some bad news; Kim died yesterday." I looked at my Mom, and replied, "Really? That's too bad." Then I walked away, with zero emotion. It bounced off me like nothing happened. It made no sense. It was like there was no more grief to give.

To say things were changing is an understatement. Everything became a physical challenge. If I jump off the garage roof, how far can I jump? Can I run all the way to school without stopping? Once that was achieved, how much faster can I do it? How many sit-ups can I do in a minute? In a row? Push-ups? Flexed arm hang?

Every year that went by, I worked on these things. I was small and wiry and becoming very athletic. Yet, it was never enough. By grade six, I could run for miles easily; I could also run fast. Doing a couple of hundred sit-ups in a row was no problem. Somehow this sense of being able to accomplish anything physical was taking root. No one encouraged me. It came from within. Push! PUSH HARDER! I hated being skinny, so I often would wear two or three sweatshirts with a t-shirt under as well. Not sure who I thought I was kidding, but it made me feel bigger. I was not small for my age, just really average.

With all the physical activity, there certainly was no fat on my frame, and at that age, a really active kid generally will not be very bulky. I wanted muscle, strength, and to feel like Superman. Like somehow, if I were big enough, I would never be bullied, picked on, or given a hard time. My neighborhood was a rougher one, so all of these things were often a part of daily life. I received my share of beatings and gave a few as well. You had to be careful. I believed that having muscle and size would be the solution. Not to mention, I figured that if I was some kind of Superman, not only would any bullying stop, but maybe my Mom would love me and be proud of me. That the girls I liked and even the ones I didn't would like me. That the guys would look up to me. That all the pain, the anger, the insecurity would all be cured, and my life would be as I had seen in some of the muscle-mags. Hanging by a pool or a beach, drinking a delicious protein drink with a lovely bikini-clad girl gazing at me adoringly! Joe Weider, the purveyor of almost all the main muscle-mags and bodybuilding equipment and supplements, knew just how to paint that picture that appealed to millions of skinny twelve-year-old boys worldwide! I ate it up. I was going to be one of those guys. Not sure how or when, but I knew it with complete certainty!

What I did not realize was this, you needed a certain genetic predisposition to look like these Mr. Universe winners. You need vast amounts of protein, thousands of hours of training, not to mention even back then, anabolic steroids were a huge part of the bodybuilding subculture. None of this would have mattered to me anyway, this knowledge. I was going to be big and strong and get the girl. All I had to do was the work, which was half the fun. I had started to enjoy pushing myself to see what I could take. There was one thing I did realize; there were NO twelve- year-old kids built like these guys. They were all grown men. I knew it would happen when I was grown. In the meantime, I would be content with pushing myself in every other way possible. After all, I wasn't normal, and I never would be again.

CHAPTER 4

"King Shit of Turd Island."

My Mom, Lucille, Lucy. Tough to write about your Mother when you know you are going to be describing some less than desirable situations.

To be frank, my Mother was the hero. Not my Dad. My Mom. She got zero credit. My Dad took the easy way out. Over the years, I have struggled with doing the very same thing. However, I was determined not to follow the same path as my Father.

Back to my Mom. She was thirty years old when my Dad took that final drive to wherever-land. Three kids. All under the age of nine. Like many women in 1974, her job was looking after us. Her formal education stopped in grade eight, and to say that it was tough getting work as an under-educated mom of three in those days is an understatement. How she kept it all together, knowing what I know now as an adult, is beyond me. She was the hero and will forever be my hero!

One of ten children and raised primarily on a farm in Saskatchewan, her childhood was tough. French was the Paulhus' first language. Like most French families of the day, Catholic. Very strict Catholics. The children all had roles on the farm, which my Grandfather ran efficiently. I barely remember him, as he passed when I was quite young. I never saw him smile, and when he was around, I was on my best behaviour. He commanded respect and had a formidable presence that could be felt. When I look at his photos now, I see that I resemble him in many ways. We both seemed to look angry all the time! My Mother told me many years later she never actually had a meaningful conversation with her Father. The children did not speak unless spoken to. There were not a lot of extras or luxuries. Mom once told me that for Christmas one year, she received a deck of cards and was very grateful for that gift.

Lucille was the second youngest and was also what was considered at the time a "bad kid." She was pretty, athletic, and charming. She liked rock and roll, especially Elvis, and she liked boys. In a sense, she was every Catholic parent's nightmare. It is hard not to laugh when I think of my Mom's wedding photos. Her Mom and Dad look more like they are at a funeral than at a wedding!

She attended a Catholic school run by nuns. By all accounts, it was not a fun place, and after the eighth grade, Lucille had decided that the working world would be a much better place for her. It's not that she was lacking in intelligence, she just could not buy into all that the Nuns were espousing. She saw that there was more to life than living in fear of hell.

My Mother never spoke much about my Dad—how they met, where, and so forth. After several talks with her and trying to get as much information as possible, I realized that it was simply too hard for her to talk about my Dad. She felt tremendous guilt for his death.

As she explained to me, "I was not nice to him Todd. I said horrible things. I was very cruel." After his death, my paternal Grandfather tried to stay in touch with us, but she did not allow this, ignoring his efforts. Her guilt was so great she later explained, she could not face his family. I grew up thinking they wanted nothing to do with me. Whenever we would speak of him, she would suffer from nightmares for days, so I realized pursuing the matter further was not fair to her. She did explain that when she met him, he and his family seemed like a breath of fresh air compared to her staunch, strict, no-fun catholic family! They drank too much, of course. They laughed; they carried on and had fun. As far as French families at the time, each family represented a different side of the proverbial coin. She was nineteen when they married, and my Mom said her parents were simply relieved to get her married off before she ended up getting pregnant.

Compared to my Maternal Grandparents, my Mom was a pussycat. That being said, she was tough as nails! Just in comparison, she was soft. She made efforts at different times to talk to me as a kid. Usually, when she had been drinking, which she was doing more and more to cope. Some of the talks were good, though. By today's standards, I was raised in an abusive home. People tend to carry that like some badge of honour these days and whine about it forever. My Mom did what she had to. I know she feels bad for much of it. To be perfectly honest, looking back, I do not know how she didn't kill all three of us! I would have.

She had found a job as a waitress at the Vendome Hotel in Downtown Winnipeg, working the evening shift. Every night as she left for work, I would watch her walk to the bus stop, my head pressed hard against the metal mesh screen of my window that overlooked the street. That screen became permanently bowed out from my head as I often fell asleep in that position sitting up. I was convinced she was never coming back, that she too would die or be killed. So, every night my mission was to stay up until she came back. I always failed.

It was not very often that my Mother had to tell us anything twice. Repercussions were swift and severe. She ran a tight ship. There are many examples. This one is a minor one. My Mom took me on a shopping excursion to the big department stores in downtown Winnipeg. Eaton's and The Bay. Walking by the toy section, I asked if I could look at toys while she shopped. The common thing in those days was to leave your kid in the toy section while you did your shopping. When she returned, I didn't want to go and proceeded to have a bit of a tantrum. She gave me one warning, and for some odd reason, I defied her. She explained calmly that I would receive a beating when we got home and dragged me off. I eventually calmed down, and the rest of the outing went really well. Fun, in fact. When we got home, she issued one order, "go to your room. I will be in there in a minute to give you your beating!" I remember thinking, "What? But everything else went so well? We had fun? Really?" A minute later, she returned to beat the tar out of me. If nothing else, my Mother meant what she said, and she was consistent! It would be a long time before I was either brave enough or stupid enough to challenge her authority outright like that again!

Considering her circumstances, her temper could have and should have been a lot worse. She had found a slightly better job waitressing closer to home in the North Ends famous Kelekis Restaurant. It had been around forever and was famous for its hotdogs and curly fries. I loved going there as the owners were always sweet to me and would usually give me something to eat. It was family-owned, and the Kelekis sisters were famous for how tough they were. North Enders are a tough lot, to begin with. My Mom endured a lot working there, but as always, she soldiered on, and I never remember her complaining. She was exhausted when she got home and still made sure that we had a decent meal before she would hide in the sanctuary of her bedroom for a while as she tried to recover. The rule was QUIET! If she went in there, we were to be quiet. Being kids, of course, we had the attention span of gnats. So, we often broke that rule, and sometimes the consequences of that were not pleasant. Linda, being the "good kid," rarely broke that or any rule. Being the only boy, the middle child, and totally screwed in the head in many ways meant that I usually was the one instigating trouble or just being a selfish little pain in the ass. On one occasion, Mom had instructed Tina and me to do the dishes after supper as she went to relax. "I do not want to hear ANY noise, understand?" We both nodded. A few minutes later, I get it into my genius brain that starting a water fight would be a great idea. Of course, it escalated. I never saw it coming. I sure felt it. All I remember was a sharp crack to the back of the head and then hitting the floor. Then my Mom's voice, "I SAID BE QUIET!" After that, I pretty much was in la-la land for a few minutes. When I regained my senses, I realized she had cracked me over the head with a pan.

There were many times when I received a well-deserved beating. There were also times when things just went too far. I am not going to go into each and every episode. It serves no purpose as it gets redundant. I will share the most painful incident. It still pains me to think about it. What it does is paints a clear picture of what I grew up with, and it can explain much of why many of my relationships over the years went the way they did.

Mom had just returned from grocery shopping. As I helped her put away the groceries, she issued a warning, "I'm going to bed, do NOT start eating all the food!" She later explained to me many years later that me being a boy, my athletic activity level was not something she understood. I was twelve years old at the time. I was growing, and I was eating more than both of my sisters and Mother combined. At that time, she thought I was simply being a selfish pig. I was just hungry. I could go through over 4 litres of milk a day, no problem at all. It was at this age I was starting to defy my Mother. So, within fifteen minutes of her going to bed, I started to eat. I never heard her behind me. The first thing I felt was a smack to the back of the head. "YOU WANT TO EAT? NOW YOU ARE GOING TO EAT!" She dragged me by the arm to the kitchen table and threw me into my chair; I was stunned. She grabbed the entire bunch of bananas (I had been eating a banana) and a giant salad bowl. She then grabbed a full box of cereal and poured the whole box and 2 litres of milk into it. She screamed, "YOU ARE GOING TO SIT THERE UNTIL YOU HAVE EATEN ALL OF IT!!!" I was crying, sobbing. She smacked me again. "EAT!"

I began to eat. I ate as much as I could, the whole time pleading and begging and saying, "I'm sorry, I'm sorry!"

She keeps screaming at me to eat. Finally, I get to a point where I know I am going to throw up. "I'm going to barf!" That was all I could get out in between sobs. She grabs the bowl and slams it into my face. "Clean it up." Then she walked away. I never felt worse about myself as I did at that moment. I felt worthless and assumed that my Mother hated me deeply. I cleaned up the mess and left the house. I went to nearby "Roxy Park," not its real name; we just called it that because it was located across from Roxy Bowling Lanes. I sat on the river bank and contemplated everything. I wanted to die. Deep in my mind, however, there was a tiny spark. A little thought. That thought was, "One day, I will be so big, so strong. No one will ever hurt me again!"

Throughout my teen years, my Mom seemed to have a mission. That mission was to ensure that I never had a big ego. On a very regular basis, she seemed to feel the need to put me in my place. Over time, this was quite damaging, and I did withdraw from most things and often stayed up late at night as I did not have the confidence to face most people.

As she liked to put it, "Who do you think you are, King Shit of Turd Island?"

CHAPTER 5

"Shoulder down."

It was the Harlem Globetrotters that introduced me to the world of basketball. Of course, I knew what basketball was, but it was not until I happened upon the Trotters on ABC's Wide World of Sports that I became aware of the absolute beauty of the sport. Unlike most Canadian boys, I never played hockey and could not skate. Even in the 1970s, hockey was an expensive sport. My Mother knew there was absolutely no way she could afford to put me in hockey, so she simply avoided the subject and did not allow me to have skates until I was eight years old. Well, by that age, most boys can skate like the wind. I was used to being one of the better athletes amongst my peers. On the ice, I was as helpless as a baby. Not to mention I have always hated the cold. I remember trying to skate as my peers whizzed by me as I hobbled around the ice, my ankles bent at a horrific angle. It didn't take long to realize this was not for me. I was so cold I could not get the laces undone and ended up walking awkwardly home several blocks from Kelvin Community Club rink to my house. I was done with hockey and skating!

As far as equipment, basketball was easy. It wasn't hard to convince my Mom to buy me my first basketball for my birthday. In my house, you received gifts on birthdays and Christmas. There was no, "Mom buy me this!" That would never fly. You wanted something; birthday or Christmas was the time. Despite not having much money, Mom was amazing at saving and budgeting. We were never spoiled, yet somehow Mom always made sure we got what we asked for on those days! The $12.99 Jelinek Basketball was an easy sell! Once I got the ball, I was determined to become the best basketball player I could. Like every physical challenge, I attacked it with tunnel vision. That ball went everywhere with me. In the springtime, I would shovel snow off of outdoor courts and shoot hoops until my hands froze. No one else my age played basketball in my hood. It was all hockey, soccer, and some football. As per my habit, I picked something unusual. I wanted to be different; in my mind, I was different! Basketball was a Junior and Senior High sport.

At the end of Grade Six, our teacher Mr. Neufeld recommended that I attend a basketball camp that Elmwood Junior High was holding. He had worked with me all year to help me build confidence. He was aware of my home life and my struggles with anger. I was thrilled when he told me about the camp! It was almost not to be, as was to become a pattern in my life, I would do my best to sabotage a positive situation as I had no skill set to deal with success. Let me explain what a positive force Mr. Neufeld was in my young life. He was to become the first of many mentors that helped me in my life and tried to steer me in the right direction! One day towards the end of the school year, Mr. Neufeld took us out to the ball field for a class softball game. As I stepped into the batter's box, I prepared myself to smack the hell out of the ball. I had been playing softball since a young age with my friends each summer in pick-up games and was pretty decent at it. Then something strange happened. First pitch, swing, and a miss. "What the hell?" I thought to myself. STRIKE TWO! Missed again. Now I was getting pissed. I gritted my teeth and steadied myself. STRIKE THREE! I walked away in total disbelief. This was NOT acceptable. There was some snickering from my friends. To me, this was a huge embarrassment. The temper began to rumble. Next time up, three pitches, three strikes. No more snickering. My classmates had seen me lose it on more than one occasion, once throwing my desk across the classroom. My last time up, they started pitching to me like they would the feeble kids in the class, trying to let me get contact on the ball. This infuriated me! Try as I might, I could not hit the damn ball! STRIKE THREE! "ARGH!!!!!" I yelled as loud as I could and threw the bat into the outfield. I sat down on the grass and did not speak for the rest of the day. No one spoke to me. At the end of the day, as school let out, Mr. Neufeld asked me to stay after school. I knew I was in trouble. After everyone had left, and no one was in the schoolyard, he said, "Todd, follow me." He grabbed a bat, ball, and a glove. We walked together back to the ball field. "Get in the batter's box Todd." "I CAN'T hit it, Mr. Neufeld!" I felt tears welling up in my eyes. He walked over to me, placed his hand on my shoulder, and quietly said, "Yes, you can, Todd, I will teach you." Every day that week, after school, he calmly and patiently taught me how to watch the ball, focus on good contact, and not try to kill it. By the end of that week, I was connecting consistently and with force. I loved him for that.

Self-sabotage. I was the master of this. Despite Mr. Neufeld's patience, I could still snap. Especially if embarrassed.

This one particular day, I was struggling with math as I often did. Math to this day is a foreign language to me, and I have no gift for it. Mr. Neufeld asked me a question. I was not paying attention and had no answer. He lightly scolded me and told me that I better start paying attention. I was embarrassed being called out like that. The temper flared.

As he walked away, I flipped him off with both hands. He turned around just at that moment. I now understand his anger, as he had made real efforts to help me, and I was basically telling him to fuck off in front of the whole class. He grabbed me, dragged me out into the hall, and threw me onto the chair that was just outside of the class.

All he said was this, "Think about what you just did, Todd, and WHO you did it to!" He could not have chosen more effective words. I completely broke down. Completely.

He came back after what seemed like an eternity. He asked me, "Why?"

I simply did not know. I could not express why I had so much anger. My big fear was that he would take away basketball camp. I asked him if I could still attend.

He answered, "Of course, but not if you lose your temper again."

I will tell you this: I never lost my temper again with Mr. Neufeld or in his class.

Elmwood High School. Grades 7 – 12. I remember walking into the gym for the first time and thought I was in heaven. It was huge! Six basketball hoops, a full-size court, and what seemed like a thousand kids all shooting hoops and running around. I felt nervous with so many kids, but this was REAL basketball, and that helped me to overcome that fear and apprehension. They began rounding us up into groups and showing us various drills: Layups, ball handling, proper shooting technique, defensive stance, and passing. I was one of the only, if not the only, kid my age that could do all of it. I could dribble with both hands, shoot layups right and left, and had decent ball control. Elmwood had a strong basketball program, and they wanted it to continue, which is why they ran the camp in the first place. They had great coaching through every grade. Two of the coaches, Mr. Korsunsky and Mr. Kelsh, were also guidance counsellors. They would be a big influence on me and did their very best to keep me out of trouble.

It was Sid Korsunsky that noticed me first. I was the only kid that could shoot a left-handed layup with proper footwork and actually using my left hand. He called me over.

"What's your name?"

I liked him immediately. He was about five foot nine, dark curly hair, athletic build, and a great 80's mustache. Coach K, as we called him, had serious fundamental skills while not being the fastest or able to jump high, he could simply outthink you, outshoot you, and he didn't make mistakes.

"Where did you learn to play, Todd? Did your Dad teach you?"

"No, I don't have a Dad, I taught myself."

"That's impressive. I will be keeping an eye out for you at tryouts, are you attending Elmwood next year?"

"Yes, I will be."

He then called over coaches Harrison and Kelsh and had me show them what I could do. I wasn't used to the attention. It was amazing. In my house, I was either ignored or being yelled at.

Basketball was very black and white for me. I loved that. You either made the shot, or you didn't. Succeed or fail. Again, that feeling from within was taking hold. If you worked hard enough, you would succeed. There was no "could" in my world. It was "would." It never bothered me to spend endless hours practicing. Even then, when I was tired and was done for the day, I had a routine I had to get perfect before I allowed myself to leave. I had to shoot a layup from both sides. Then hit shots from every hash mark around the key. Then a shot from each baseline. A foul shot and a three-pointer. All shots not only had to go in but the ball also was not allowed to touch the rim! Each shot had to be a perfect "swish." This often resulted in an extra hour of this drill until it went perfect. Only then did I allow myself to leave. What this did was make me very sound in my basic skills. I could shoot from anywhere. Because I dribbled that ball everywhere I went, my ball handling was good. I also ran almost everywhere, so I didn't often fatigue. I was not afraid of hard work. It was my sanity. Black and white. In a world where I felt "different," where I felt I had no control, basketball was my sanity.

Confidence was the issue. While my skill set was very developed, games were an entirely different matter—even scrimmages in practice or one-on-one drills. I simply did not have the confidence to shoot even when the opportunity was there. In one-on-one drills, I would not attack the basket or create opportunities to score. Instead, I would let my opponent drive me away from the hoop only to put up a haphazard off-balance shot. I would not square up for fear of having my shot blocked.

Coach K changed that for me. It was so simple, such an easy lesson. It entirely changed my game, and as a result, I started to find a little bit of confidence. I was playing one-on-one with a kid one grade above me. I still remember his name, Steve Sacher. I had the ball, and as per usual, I let Steve force me away from the basket, and I threw some ugly ass shot. Coach K was watching. "TODD! Why are you letting him force you away like that? Drive to the basket, shoulder down, and blow by him! Let me show you." Coach shuffled over; he never walked; he shuffled. He was known for it. In the mornings before school, Coach K would open up the gym for any of us that wanted to free scrimmage. We could always hear the shuffle before we saw him. Coach K was cool.

"Watch." he instructed.

Steven got in a defensive position.

Coach threw a fake left at him, dropped his shoulder, went right, and blew by Steve like he wasn't there for an easy layup.

"See? Shoulder down. Take the space. Own it. It's your space. Give the opponent no chance. We both know you can go right or left, so he has to respect that. You can throw a fake or two. All you have to do is make him move slightly, then drop the shoulder and blow by him. Boom! Lay up!"

Coach threw me the ball. This time, I threw a couple of fakes, made Steve fall for one, and I dropped my shoulder and blew by him for an easy layup. I was shocked. It worked. I tried it again. Layup. Easy. The next time I got Steve backpedaling, and then I stopped suddenly and pulled up for an easy little jump shot. SWISH! I looked at Coach; he was smiling this big smile. I was smiling as well. It was like I had discovered gold or uranium or something. After I beat Steve, Coach called me over. "Todd, let me explain something to you. Your fundamental skills are great. You are quick. You can shoot, go left or right. You should be beating guys all the time. Be confident. If the shot is there, take it! No one will get mad at you. What's the worst that could happen? You miss? Big deal. Larry Bird misses. It's part of the game. Take the shot. Drive the lane. Make them pay. Remember, shoulder down!"

It did not take long for me to become one of the best one-on-one players in the school. I would play against anyone. Senior high guys, coaches, teammates. Anyone. I loved playing against the better older guys as it made me play better and harder and raise the level of my game. That advice has served me very well over the years.

Many years later, as I sat in a jail cell, it was Coach K's voice that I would hear in my head quietly repeating, "Shoulder down Todd, shoulder down."

CHAPTER 6

"OOK EM!!!"

While basketball may have been my first athletic love, it was certainly not the last. It seemed I was always looking for new ways to both challenge and punish myself physically and mentally. You may ask why I say mentally? Well, I soon discovered that athletic excellence was not only a test of physical strength and endurance but was, in fact, much more of a mental test. It was the brain that made the decision to forge ahead through pain and discomfort, not to mention the emotional aspect, confidence on a given day, mood, and the ability to control one's emotions. Those that could control the mind and emotional state were the ones that could get the absolute most out of their bodies. While my mental state in my everyday life was often a complete mess, when it came to focusing on an athletic event, I could push everything else out of my mind. In fact, the harder the task, the better I liked it!

Enter BOXING! Sports that were a test of toughness and strength always appealed to me. Growing up in the '70s and '80s was an amazing time in the boxing world. There was the greatest "Ali" that eclipsed everyone in the boxing universe. Let's not forget there were Joe Frazier, George Foreman, Ken Norton, Larry Holmes, Thomas "Hitman" Hearns, "Marvelous" Marvin Hagler, and "Sugar" Ray Leonard, to name but a few. There were great fights to be seen on television on a regular basis. The funny thing was, it was a fictional character that inspired me to take those first tentative steps into the world of pugilism! None other than "Rocky Balboa"! It's funny to think of now, but that story of the everyman, a guy from the streets that no one expected to ever accomplish anything, well that hit home with me.

Rocky 3 came out in the theatres the summer I was 13 years old. It was a blockbuster! The movies were a great childhood escape for me. Having seen Rocky and Rocky 2 on TV, I was thrilled when the third installment came out. Fighting against an unbeatable foe in the form of "Clubber Lang," very aptly played by a young and very raw Mr. T (before he became the homogenized caricature of himself in later years), had me on the edge of my seat! What really stood out was that Rocky got absolutely punished by Clubber in their first fight and found the intestinal fortitude to fight him a second time. He had to admit to not only himself that he was scared, but he also had to admit it to his wife, Adrianne. That scene really hit a chord with me. Accepting a challenge, facing a fear, that impressed me a great deal. By the end of that movie, when Rocky triumphed, I was in tears. I watched that movie three times in a row that day. I also came back the next week and watched it again. Then the decision was made, I was going to box, I was going to fight!!!

Being a gritty neighborhood, Elmwood, of course, had a boxing club, and it was right out of a Hollywood Movie! It was a 10- minute run from my house, and of course, I knew this because I ran everywhere. Housed in an old Fire Hall, it was very intimidating. So much so that I went there every day for a week before mustering up the courage to actually step inside. Each day I would run there and peer inside the dirty and stained window next to the entrance that was in the back of the building. Rough-looking young men would come and go as I would stare in awe. They looked like gladiators, often with black eyes, swollen lips, and various cuts and bloodstains. It was terrifying! The challenge was in conquering the fear.

Finally, and while definitely feeling like puking, I walked through that back door. The first thing that hit you as you entered the old Hall was the smell. It really hit you like a stiff jab! Blood, sweat, and humidity filled your nostrils as soon as you crossed that threshold into the gym area. Then it was the noise. Grunting, thudding of heavy bags, coaches shouting instructions, as well as the sound of heavy blows being landed during the countless sparring sessions that went on almost continually. Until you have been that close to a boxing ring during a fight, there is simply no way to comprehend the animal ferocity as well as the beauty of movement and executed skill. It is a surreal experience.

After what seemed like an eternity, I asked a young man who was shadow boxing who I needed to speak to about becoming a fighter. He looked at my less than formidable 115lb frame, chuckled, and said, "Eddie," pointing to a solidly built man in his 40's working the hand pads with a young fighter on the other side of the gym. I would later learn his full name was Eddie Yaremchuk. CRACK!!! Each time the young fighter unleashed a lighting quick blow, it sounded like the crack of a whip combined with thunder as the punches were caught skillfully by Eddie into those hand pads. I remember thinking, "how is that not breaking his hands?"

Finally, a voice yelled out "TIME!" and the young man's assault on the hand pads stopped.

The fighter that was working with Eddie saw me standing behind him and pointed to me. Eddie turned around. Man, he looked tough. He was built like a cement block. His face did not hide the many blows he had taken over the years. He looked at me and simply said, "What you want, kid?"

I started to stammer, "H-how much to join the g-gym?"

He smiled and looked me up and down. "You want to box, kid?"

I simply nodded.

"Ten bucks, make sure you show up with a mouthguard and hand wraps. Go to Athlete's Wear. They sell them. Come back tomorrow at 5:00 pm. Understand?

Again, I nodded.

The next day I showed up promptly at 5:00 pm with a crumpled ten-dollar bill. I had no money for the mouth guard or hand wraps. I was lucky that I had ten bucks at the time! I walked up to Eddie as he was wrapping the hands of a wiry-looking fighter. "I brought the ten bucks, Eddie!" He looked at me for a second, and I guess he did not remember me from the previous day. "Oh yeah, the kid wants to box. Where's your hand wraps and mouthguard?" I sheepishly looked down. Eddie had seen this very scene play out many, many times over the years. Boxing was his love, his way of giving back, teaching. It was NOT about money. He called out across the gym, "JIMMY! Get this kid some hand wraps and get him going. He wants to be a fighter! What's your name, kid?" I sputtered, "Todd." "Well, Todd, you pay me when you can for those wraps, OK? Jimmy, wrap this kid's hands and work with him, OK?" Eddie then pocketed the ten-dollar bill.

I will never forget the first time I saw Jimmy Saunders, who was now standing next to Eddie, holding a brand-new pair of hand wraps. He was a bear of a man. Wearing his hair in a perfectly trimmed crew cut (I was to learn he had spent many years as a barber), with an impossibly thick neck and barrel chest, he looked like every B

Hollywood Movie's version of an ex-boxer. Later I had learned his nickname was "Babyface" despite the fact that he looked like you could count the number of fights he had by his battle scars. His eyes, however, were gentle, kind even. "C'mon, kid." He put his huge meat hook of a hand on my shoulder and guided me over to a chair, and sat me down. "Give me your hand." He then carefully began wrapping my hands with the new hand wraps, which looked funny in comparison to all the other guy's hand wraps in the gym. Mine was so white and clean-looking. They did not stay that way for long.

After my hands were tightly wrapped up, he motioned me to follow him to a corner of the gym that had a mirror in it. He very patiently began to show me the basics. First, it was how to stand, where to keep your hands, then it was two punches. Left jab, straight right. Over and over and over. Left jab, straight right. Slowly at first, he showed me meticulously. If my hands were out of position, he corrected me. If I was off-balance, he would give me a light punch to the arm that showed me how easily you could get knocked down even from a blow that otherwise could not hurt you!

The next day, I was in shock at how sore I was. Was I an athlete after all? What I did not take into consideration was the fact that I was now using different muscles in different ways than they were used to being used. My arms were used to shooting a basketball over and over. They were NOT used to firing punches for three minutes at a time without rest. I could feel everything: my shoulders, arms, back, chest were all on fire with the slightest movement. I loved it. No matter how much it hurt, I was going back. Each day, Jimmy would show me something new. Or add an exercise. Every workout started the same for all of us—three rounds of shadow boxing in the ring. Quite a sight it was. Sometimes there could be ten or more of us all fighting invisible opponents at once. Bobbing and weaving, dancing around the ring all while firing punches. You had to watch yourself if it was crowded. If you weren't paying attention, you could end up on the wrong end of one of those shots!

As my technique improved, Jimmy would show me new skills in how to slip and block punches. Intricate combinations. Always working at increasing hand speed. How to skip rope properly. The double-ended bag that could smash you in the face if you were too slow or not focused. Then there was my favorite, the speed bag! There was nothing so satisfying as getting a good rhythm going on the speed bag. It sounded like a drum, and of course, every boxing movie worth its salt showed a fighter working the speed bag. I would do countless rounds on it, pushing myself to hit it faster and faster!

At the end of each workout, Jimmy would take me through various old-school calisthenics. Tons of push-ups, sit-ups off the end of a table as Jimmy held my legs in place, neck bridges to handle punches better. Jimmy was in his 50's and would do every exercise I did, set for set and for more reps. He was strong as a bull. He no longer had the fast hands of a young fighter, but if Jimmy decided to do a few rounds on the heavy bag, you almost felt sorry for the bag! Jimmy had a left hook that would probably dent a truck. WAP!! THUD!! Every time he launched that hook, and believe me launched is the best way to describe it; you would hear the impact no matter where you were in the gym. That power impressed me, and I did my best to learn from Jimmy and emulate him the best I could.

One day we were working on the hand pads together. Three-minute rounds always. For the last 30 seconds of each round, Jimmy would have me fire off only two punches as rapidly as I could over and over until the round ended. Basically, a final flurry at the end of the round when you are tired. It was always a straight right and a left hook. Two power bombs designed to do one thing, knock your opponent into oblivion. Jimmy would shout out, "RIGHT! OOK EM (ook em was Jimmy's way of saying hook him)!!! RIGHT! OOK EM!" I would fire these shots off as fast and as hard as I could, trying my best to decimate my imaginary foe! Well, on this particular day, my right hand was off target, and I cracked Jimmy square in the jaw! I promptly dropped both hands and exclaimed, "GEEZ JIMMY, I'M SORRY! ARE YOU OK?" Without blinking, dropping the hand pads, or missing a beat, he shouted, "OOK EM!"

It was at that moment I learned two things, Jimmy was the toughest person I had met in my life, and I had better work harder!

CHAPTER 7

"You SHOULD be scared, I would be!"

If you have never stepped into a boxing ring, never sparred, never fought, then I do not know if you can fully appreciate why boxing is referred to as "the sweet science." It is truly a science. It is physics; it is the science of the mind and the body working synergistically. It is also primal and vicious, and animalistic in every sense of the word. It takes a fine athlete that has been blessed with certain physical, genetic traits such as quickness, power, stamina, and strength. Not to mention their body's ability to absorb punishment. Some people simply get knocked out easily; you can't TRAIN for that. As quick as Ali was, he could also take tremendous punishment. Don't believe me? Watch his fight with Foreman. Foreman was a monster, and next to perhaps only Earnie Shavers, he was probably the second hardest puncher of all time. Ali LET Foreman beat on him for eight rounds until George was so tired Ali threw a quick combination, and that was it for George. Think about that for a second. He LET Foreman beat on his head, arms, shoulders, and body for almost eight whole rounds. Literally hundreds of bone-breaking punches! The power in those punches would have pretty much-killed anyone else. Ali was not an ordinary man. Ali simply absorbed them, taunting George the whole time. That can't be taught or trained for.

The single most important trait that seemed to be common to every great fighter I have ever seen was one that the average person may never consider. The truly great fighters were not only amazing athletes that could take tremendous physical punishment, they were something else entirely. They were in every sense of the word "killers." When a real fighter gets you in trouble, you better hope to hell the ref is there close by and stops the fight because one of these guys will punch your head off. They have an extra switch, an extra gear, they smell blood, and you are done. There is not necessarily anger in what they do. In reality, there is no anger. It is not unlike a shark with an injured, bloodied fish. They finish it. No ands, ifs, or buts. They can hug you after, shake your hand, be civil, and all that stuff you see in post-fight interviews. However, when you are in their jungle, you are prey. Kill or be killed. Good night Irene!

I was a good athlete. Quick and coordinated and not afraid of hard work. My balance was decent, and for my size, I could hit quite hard. My straight right was my best punch, and I would later learn it could inflict some damage! What I was not was what I really needed to be, and that held me back. Try as I might, I did not have that "killer edge!" Do not get me wrong, I will defend myself. In my life, I have been in more than one ugly physical altercation. When it came to boxing, though, I loved the training. I would train all day. After a while, they gave me a key and would let me stay as late as I wanted. I would simply keep training after everyone else wanted to leave.

Sparring was another thing, though. I HATED sparring for a couple of reasons. When I started boxing, there was only one other kid, named Jeff, close to me in age at the club. He was two years older than me, 6 inches taller, and at least 50 lbs heavier. That was who I had to spar with. It didn't end there. He was a bully. When we sparred, I tried to work on whatever skill they wanted me to work on. Not him. He would simply do his best to knock my head off. It was boxing, after all, and our club was a tough one. Sparring sessions could be intense, bloody affairs. They didn't encourage his brutality, but at the same time, I had to learn to survive in the ring.

They let that evolve, and it certainly was a motivation for me to train harder. So, for the first three months or so, I was literally getting beaten up two-four times a week. Not much fun, but I stuck it out, determined to get the better of this 15-year-old version of Baby Huey. Every day that I ran to the gym, I would be hoping I would not see Jeff's stepdad's car in the parking lot. If it was there, I knew there was a pretty good chance I might be taking a beating that day! As with most things in my life, I did not let that stop me. No point in lying; I was scared of Jeff. That fear had to be dealt with, conquered. After each sparring session, he would gloat, always had a smart-ass comment directed at me. Deep inside, I would hear that voice. There was that spark. Coach K whispering, "Shoulder down, Todd. Shoulder down, own the space, make it yours!" My day would come.

My personal philosophy was reinforced during this time. That being, if you were willing to put in the physical work and your focus was in place, then any goal was obtainable. Sadly, I did not see the correlation between this outlook and making it pertain to achieving goals in everyday life, which for me was often filled with self-hate, insecurities, and fear. In the gym, it was like I had blinders on, and I had the ability to shut everything negative out of my brain. I was improving and gaining strength and endurance, as well as becoming quite adept at throwing fast and complex punch combinations. In time, the challenges in the gym were not enough, and I started doing intense road work that consisted of running from my house to downtown Winnipeg (several miles). Once Downtown, I would run to the Holiday Towers Apartment Complex and run up the stairs, which were 26 stories tall. Then I would run down the stairs and back home. When I reached the last block, I would sprint all out so that when I got to our house, I would totally collapse, lying on the grass waiting for my breathing to return to normal. The more it hurt at the end of that run, the greater the sense of accomplishment! Black and white. It all made sense. These little victories gave me purpose and kept me going!

My relationship with Jimmy grew. He took me into his world. Often, when he could, he would stay late with me in the gym. He would work with me until I simply could no longer go on. More often than not, I would walk home with him after. We lived in the same area. It was a bit out of my way, but hearing his boxing stories made it well worth it. He had fought Floyd Patterson as an Amateur. He won a medal in the Common Wealth Games. He had been the Canadian Heavyweight Champion. He let me see all his boxing memorabilia. I have always loved history, and I loved pouring over old scrapbooks and newspaper clippings with him. Looking at these old photos taught me how he got the nickname "Babyface." Before the countless blows and Father Time had taken their toll, Jimmy had, in fact, had a babyface. As a young man, he always smiled in photos, and you would never know by looking at him that he had a left hook that could knock you senseless in very short order!

Finally, the day came that I had not really given much thought to. I was sitting, wrapping my hands with my now bloodstained wraps. Thinking about the training I was about to undergo when Eddie came over to me and sat down next to me on the sit-up table. "Hey kid, we have a tournament in two weeks. I got you a fight. You will have to get your Mom to sign a release form. I guess he could see the fear in my eyes. With a big slap on my shoulder, he chuckled, "Don't worry, kid, you will be fine, you're ready!" I gulped and felt the blood drain from my face. A fight? A real fight? In front of people? Visions of a 13-year-old version of Clubber Lang appeared in my mind. I didn't think I was ready. Not to mention, I had never actually told my Mom I was boxing. Now I had to get permission. The tournament was to take place in a small town in Saskatchewan, Carnduff, I believe it was called. We would all be going in a big van. "Aw damn." I thought to myself.

It took several days for me to gather up the guts to tell my Mom about boxing and the tournament. I had no idea what to expect, other than a bad reaction. Her reaction was almost a non–reaction. All she said was, "You want to box? Fine. Do not come crying to me with black eyes and bloody noses." She then signed the release form and handed it back to me. She had a slight smile as she did so, which worried me. Perhaps part of me wanted her to say no. That was the coward in me. I would have to do it. Conquer the fear. It was not negotiable.

The days flew by. Before I could fully grasp what I actually was doing, we were all at the club loading our gear into a large van/bus early on a July Saturday morning. The drive from Winnipeg to Carnduff was about four hours. My family did not own a car since Dad passed. Four hours was a long drive for me. What made it worse was the feeling of impending doom. I felt like a gladiator being led out to his fate in the coliseum. At 13, many of us have ways of taking situations and making them very dramatic. I was no different, and all I could think of was that I was about to get beat up, far from home, in front of a crowd of people. I wanted to throw up. I don't think I said anything the whole drive there. Jimmy sat next to me. He knew what was going on in my head but didn't say a word. He picked his spot. He knew what to say and when to say it. When it turned out to be as he was wrapping my hands for my fight, my opponent was a 13-year-old kid named Jason Greenway. It was his first fight as well. We were bantamweights.

Finally, Jimmy spoke, "Are you scared?"

I nodded yes.

"Good! You SHOULD be scared. I would be!" I couldn't believe what I was hearing. He went on, "Fights are scary. Especially the first one." He continued to carefully wrap my hands and then asked, "That big dumb kid you spar with, Jeff? That kid probably weighs 150-160lbs! Man, he laid some beatings on you! You never gave up, though. He never knocked you out. Isn't that something? Kid that big couldn't knock you out!"

I listened intently, blocking out every other sound. Jeff had not been coming to the gym as regularly, and when we sparred, he was starting to get frustrated. He was still beating me, but not nearly as badly. I was getting good. He couldn't always catch me. He was slow, and he didn't train hard. He would get tired, and I was getting to the point where I could tag him. He was only beating me with size at this point. "Todd, you will fight better being a bit scared. It's natural. Today you are fighting a kid YOUR SIZE! You are going to fight as hard as you can! In fact, when the bell goes, and you walk out into the middle of the ring, you are going fire off that big straight right hand! You try and take his head off!"

Jimmy was smiling, animated. He had me practice walking straight forward and throwing that lead right. "Jimmy, you really think I can knock him out with the first punch?" He put his big paw on my shoulder and quietly said, "Never know, sometimes you get lucky!" With that, the tension was broken, we both busted out laughing. He had put everything in perspective. I was stilled scared, but I had realized that whatever this kid Jason could dish out would be nothing worse than what I had endured every week for months!

The time came to walk to the ring. The tunnel vision kicked in. I was wearing blue and gold trunks that said "Pan Am Boxing Club on them, with a white tank top. I heard nothing. The focus was there. We were led to the center of the ring. To my surprise, my opponent was not a pint-sized Clubber Lang, but a kid MY SIZE that looked every bit the beginner that I was. I felt a small amount of relief. The pre-fight instructions could have been in Russian. I didn't hear a word. We just stared at each other. They made us touch gloves, and then we went back to our respective corners. Jimmy leaned in, "Go get him! You throw that big right! You go get him!"

DING-DING!!! Round one. I met my opponent in the middle of the ring and fired that right hand. WOOOSH! All it connected with was air. My reward was a sharp jab to the chin. That was all I needed. The fear left, the crowd vanished. It was this kid, Jason, and myself. Here we go. Back and forth it went. We were evenly matched, with me being slightly quicker. I started to time him a bit. When he jabbed, he would drop his right hand leaving his head exposed—a big mistake. Whenever I did that in training, my reward was a right hand from Jimmy, hard enough to make me aware of how dangerous it was to drop your hands at any time! The next time he threw that jab, I slipped it and threw the right as hard as I could, and it tagged him square on the button! Down he went!

The next thing I knew, the ref was ushering me to a neutral corner. I wasn't clear as to what had happened until the ref went over to Jason and began a count. "HOLY CRAP!!!" I thought to myself, "I dropped him!" Jason popped up almost right away. The ref wiped off his gloves and made sure he was ok to continue.

Then I made a BIG mistake. Instead of pouncing on him, I went right back into the rhythm of the fight. I let him fight his way back. What was lacking was that killer instinct. If I had swarmed him, got him in trouble, the fight would have been stopped.

DING, DING!

Back in the corner with Jimmy, "GREAT PUNCH! WHY DID YOU LET HIM OFF THE HOOK? Go out there and take his head off! RIGHT HAND AND THEN OOK EM! DON'T BE SO DAMN HAPPY WITH YOURSELF!!!

DING-DING! Round two.

What ensued was brutal. I am quite sure whatever Jason's corner told him lit a fire underneath him, and we spent that next round absolutely tearing into each other—right in the middle of the ring, pouring it on toe to toe. I found out later many felt we had the fight of the tournament. We were very evenly matched.

DING-DING!

Back to my stool with Jimmy. "Jimmy, is my nose bleeding?" I had never had a nosebleed in my life and was wondering if today was the day.

He ignored my question and told me what I needed to hear, "LAST ROUND! IT'S REALLY CLOSE, AND WE ARE IN HIS TOWN. I THINK RIGHT NOW YOU GUYS ARE EVEN. HE WON THAT ROUND. WITH THE KNOCKDOWN, IT'S PROBABLY A DRAW!!! GO GET IT!!!

He rinsed off my mouthpiece and put it in my mouth.

DING-DING!

Round three. Jason was bleeding. We touched gloves and started trying to take each other out. I missed with a big right hand and

CRACK!!! I felt my head snap back viciously from a left hook. It was the only time I heard the crowd, and what I heard was OHHHHHHHH! Not good. Then something strange happened, I got tired. I was having trouble holding my guard up. We continued to trade shots. I was not quitting by any stretch. I was giving everything I had. Every bit of anger I had, all the pain, came out of me in those last couple of minutes. I didn't care if he killed me. I was not quitting. I was not going down.

DING-DING.

Fight over. We hugged. His face looked like he had been through a meat grinder. They announced the decision. He won by split decision, one point. I didn't care. I was elated. I had emptied myself completely. I felt tears stream down my face. I wasn't sobbing. It was just a release.

Jimmy hugged me. "Attaboy! I'm proud of you! Go shower. Clean up." I couldn't look at him. Those words meant everything to me.

"Look at me, Todd!" I did.

"Your nose is bleeding now!" We both burst out laughing!!!

I wasn't prepared for the sight that greeted me in the locker room mirror. I am still amazed my nose wasn't broken. It bled all right. My white tank top was now crimson. I had a cut over one eye. My mouth was swollen. I had the tar beaten out of me, and I was happy. I took the longest shower I had ever taken in my life. I stood there, thinking of everything, all the pain, the beatings from Jeff in the ring. I thought of my Dad and broke down. I am glad no one was there. As loud as I could with my busted-up mouth, I screamed as loud as I could, "I'M NOT A LOSER!!!"

I would never lose another fight. Hell, that loss was the biggest win in my life to that point.

CHAPTER 8

"Fuck you, Jeff!"

In some regards, an argument can be made that boxing is a microcosm of society as a whole. There are victories, losses, justices, and injustices. Every once in a while, karma will make its presence known. This chapter is kind of a postscript to Chapter 7.

As in society, a gym (whether it be a boxing, MMA, or weightlifting gym) will have many different types of people and personalities. In our little gym, we had one individual that thought he was the second coming of none other than Muhammed Ali himself. His name was Shawn. He was young and fast. Talented for sure. He definitely was a good amateur but nowhere near as good as he thought he was. I was happy that I was never put in the ring with him as he would have tortured me. He was in his early 20's, however, he would victimize anyone he was capable of dominating, no matter their age or skill level. He would showboat, gloat, and would punish those that he could. He did not care what your skill level was, and he would not pull back to half speed or follow instructions of any kind from the coaches. He was not well-liked by anyone in the gym, winning record or not. Enter KARMA. As was sometimes the case, we would have various Pro's training in our club if they were in town for a fight.

On this one occasion, a tough middleweight pro from Detroit was in town for a fight and was spending a week or so at our gym completing his final prep and keeping his reflexes sharp. He decided to do some "light sparring" and asked Eddie if Shawn could go a few rounds with him. Eddie smiled and said, "Sure."

Eddie had been around a long time and knew what was going to happen. Today, Shawn would go to school. As they climbed into the ring, the Pro called across to Shawn, "We are going easy. I'm not wearing headgear and not using a mouthguard. Just working on timing, ok?" Shawn nodded, and Eddie called, "TIME!" They started to circle one another. The Pro was doing as he said, going easy and throwing light punches. To this day, I do not know if Shawn was stupid, that arrogant, or really believed he was that good! As per his habit, Shawn ignored what he was supposed to be doing and started throwing punches with bad intentions at the Pro. Everyone in the gym at the time stopped to watch, as we all had a feeling what was going to happen.

The Pro kept warning him, "Go, easy man, go easy!" to no avail.

"TIME" yelled Eddie.

The Pro came over to Eddie and said, "What the fuck is wrong with your boy? Tell him to back off, or I will tune him up!"

Eddie smiled and quietly uttered, "Do it, man. Take him out"

The Pro nodded and started chuckling. He ducked through the ropes and challenged Shawn, "C'mon superstar, let's do this!" His whole demeanor changed. His movements resembled a jungle cat ready to pounce. Shawn threw a quick jab. He slipped it easily and landed a forceful four-punch combination that was so fast and brutal that everyone in the gym went "oooooooooohhh" at once! Shawn hit the canvas and sat there with a stunned expression on his face. The Pro simply looked at him, "Get up, superstar, c'mon, we are having fun now." He had such a cool way of speaking, and he was a killer. Shawn glanced over to Eddie. Not sure if he was expecting help, but all he received from Eddie was two words, "Get up." He got up, and the Pro started laughing and jive-talking as he landed jab after jab. He was lighting quick, but what really stood out was the power. I saw close-up the difference between a good amateur and a good pro. No comparison. The Pro simply dictated EVERYTHING that happened in the ring—slipping punches easily and landing whenever and wherever he wanted to. He literally was taking Shawn apart and giving him a taste of his own medicine ten-fold. The worst was the body shots. There is nothing that hurts worse than a solid body shot, and Shawn went down twice from them. Each time Eddie would say, "Get up." And the onslaught would continue. Finally, when the Pro had enough of this cat and mouse, he launched into a beautiful and savage combination and left Shawn a bloody quivering heap on the canvas. That was the last time anyone ever saw Shawn in our gym, and he was not missed.

Ah, Jeffrey.

After my fight, I kept going to the gym. Training and learning. Getting faster and stronger. Jeff began to fall off the map. He wasn't coming very much at all. Then he vanished for a few months. One day in November, he showed up. I had grown a couple of inches, and while not near as big as Jeff, he did not tower over me as he once had. Jimmy called me over after noticing Jeff in the gym. Jimmy never liked Jeff, as Jimmy HATED bullies. If you were bigger or more advanced, you were not supposed to beat the crap out of those smaller or less skilled. We were supposed to help each other. Sometimes sparring got out of hand, as was the nature of this sport, but that was more the exception, and the coaches tried to match us evenly as possible. "Todd, it's time you tuned up fat ass over there!" Jimmy said in a low menacing voice. "Think I can, Jimmy?" I asked. Jimmy didn't answer. He called over to Jeff, "Jeff, spar, let's go!" As we got in the ring, Jeff looked at me with his cocky grin. I wasn't smiling. "TIME!" called Jimmy. I started moving around the ring easily. Jeff looked slow and cumbersome. I was no longer afraid. I made him chase me. He hadn't been training, and within 30 seconds, he was open-mouth breathing. He was tired. Jimmy simply shouted instructions, and I followed them. "JAB IM!" he called out. I began snapping jabs, and to my delight, they were finding their target easily. When Jeff tried to tie me up, Jimmy would call out "break," and I would make Jeff chase me more. He would try hitting me with slow, awkward shots, and I WOULD MAKE HIM PAY! The body shots were killing him. Jimmy started calling out various combinations. After the third one, Jeff fell with a thud. He was bleeding from the nose and could not catch his breath. I walked over to him, leaned over, and quietly said, "Fuck-you, Jeff!" That was the last time I saw him.

CHAPTER 9

"You have a Dad!"

I suppose in the long run knowing the truth is better than living your life with false realities. In this case, finding out the truth about my Dad only confused me further about who I was in the first place.

It was probably not much more than a year after my Dad took his life that my mother started "seeing" someone. I still remember meeting "Neil" for the first time at my Mom's pre-game meeting she held with us before he arrived. We were not to bug him and so on and that we better listen to her while he was visiting.

Enter Neil. He was a big man, close to six feet tall and a solid 190lbs. Compared to my Dad, he was massive. Andy was only about five foot nine and 150lbs at the very most, and that's being generous. Neil had a deep voice, and I was pretty much in awe of him right away. Being kids and curious, we asked all kinds of questions of him. I'm pretty sure I was the biggest pain and asked the most. His answers were never serious. When I asked him where he lived, his answer was, "In a treehouse," and so forth. Never a straight answer. His visits started to become a regular thing, as did his phone calls.

My Mom and Neil would always hang out in the living room each time he visited and, a pretty short while after, retire to her bedroom. We would always get the warning to leave them alone and not to come to the door unless one of us was dying. We routinely ignored that and would be banging on her door to resolve our sibling squabbles. I can only imagine how much that would rain on their parade, so to speak. Neil never spent the night, ever. He made no effort to connect with any of us in any way, and any conversations we had were pretty brief. He was pretty intimidating, not mean or anything. He just didn't pay much attention to us. I would ask my Mom if she was going to marry Neil, and that was a question that was pretty much brushed off. After a while, I stopped asking. This pattern of Neil visiting went on for years, and he became part of the routine of our household. Only once did I cross him in any way. I was arguing with my Mom about something stupid, and he gave me a warning to listen. I don't know what got into me other than I was pretty mad and didn't have much respect for him as he had never acted like he gave a damn about any of us. So, I told him I didn't have to listen to him. The backhand across the head told me otherwise, and it sent me sailing. "Don't ever talk back to me, boy," was all he said. I would never forget that backhand.

Not long after that incident, my Mom said she wanted to talk to me. I was 11 years old at the time. She asked me to sit down. I remember thinking it must be something big. Or that I was in trouble. She took a deep breath and asked, "Todd, what do you think of Neil?"

I wasn't sure what she meant. He had barely acknowledged my existence. What was I supposed to think of him? "He's ok, I guess." was all I could come up with.

She continued, "I have to tell you something about your Dad. Andy was not your father. Neil is your biological father. I had an affair, and I became pregnant as a result with you. After you were born, Andy and I tried to work things out. We stayed together, and Tina was born. So, you have a Dad. Neil is your Dad." Stunned does not come even close to describing what I felt at that moment. Then I felt the anger welling up. I started screaming at my Mom for the first time in my life! I didn't care if she beat me. "HOW COULD YOU DO THAT TO DAD! YOU CHEATED ON HIM!" Then I asked, "Did he know? Did he know I wasn't his son?" "Yes, he knew. I told him." she answered. She did her best to calm me down. After all, I had a dad; this was a good thing, right? I tried to see her point. I could tell she felt terrible. Many years later, I asked her why she told me. Her reply was that she could see I wanted a father so bad, she thought I should know. Maybe she thought Neil would step up and actually be more than a sperm donor. This knowledge did one thing for me at that point in my life. It destroyed my reality.

For the next little while, when Neil would visit, I tried to bond with him. I tried calling him Dad. My Mom had told him I knew the truth. This did not bring him any closer to me on any level. He was there to see my Mom. He said he loved her. What his true feelings were, I will never know. He did not have any interest in me whatsoever. Later he would fear me. Later I would hold all the cards. I would have the power to destroy his life, but that was years away. At this point, I was an 11-

year-old kid that was trying to figure out why my "Dad" acted like I did not exist.

As I tried to process everything, I came to my own conclusions. I now blamed myself for Andy's death, feeling that me being the son of another man must have torn him apart. I was his only "son," after all, born on his birthday, and yet I wasn't really "his." Yet, he treated me amazingly.

It did not make sense. In my mind, it was the main reason he killed himself. I'm sure it played a part. I figured I must be pretty useless. My own father that I saw every week, would barely talk to me. He never did anything with me, never tried to be a dad, despite my constant asking to spend time with him. I had started to think that Mom hated me as well; after all, I was an "accident," a bastard. I wasn't supposed to even be there. This newfound knowledge that I was supposed to be happy about made me feel worse than ever.

What I did not know was this, Neil was still married, and I had two brothers. My day would come.

CHAPTER 10

"How much do you think you are worth?"

As much as the black and white world of athletics made sense to me, in my personal life, the real world was a complete and total disaster. Many that knew me from the age of 13 – 20 may have described me as arrogant and possibly conceited. What I ACTUALLY was, well, it was as far away from arrogant as you could be. Anything I showed on the outside was complete and total self-preservation. As I stated earlier, my Mom is a hero to me, dealing with everything she did as well as she did.

That being said, after the age of 12, she had no idea what to do with me. Much of that was me being a male. I think she harboured a certain distrust for all males on some level. Understandably so. Growing up in a house with only females and from certain things I witnessed growing up, I share that distrust of most males. I have always found it easier to communicate with women. My Mom was simply at a loss with me. She could not understand how my mind functioned and why boys did the stupid things they did. Add in that I was starting to rebel, had all kinds of anger issues, and started to test her. This was a recipe for disaster! I used to tell my friends that in her eyes, I was "the cause of all the world's problems." I was starting not to care. This is always bad, but especially with youth. I started to steal from her and sometimes from my older sister.

To this day, I am ashamed of this. I justified it at the time by telling myself that they both hated me. There was definitely truth to that with my older sister. Linda was going through her own personal hell at school with her peers, and I certainly did nothing to endear myself to her. From the time I was 13 until I was in my early twenties she did not really talk to me and referred to me only as "asshole."

I thought she was cold, mean. There was no way I could understand any of the things she was going through. When our Dad died, never once did I see her shed a tear. I was to learn later what an amazing and strong person she was and is. Linda never let us see her cry because she was protecting Mom.

While I was losing my mind, Linda felt Mom had enough to deal with and did not want to burden her further. Everything Linda did, she did herself. She finished high school with high grades, worked, and put herself through University. She has a great career in the dental industry and has traveled the world. My big sister is tough. I admire her and love her very much. I wish I had paid closer attention to the example of true strength and fortitude she displayed when we were kids.

School was becoming an issue. Junior High and High School can be tough for many kids. I simply did not have the confidence needed to be a success. Even when I did something well, I wasn't sure how to process it or feel that it was deserved. In my mind, it was simpler not to go. This, of course, caused all kinds of problems. The biggest for me was sports. If you did not attend, you were not allowed to play sports. Coach K did everything he could to try and help me, as did Coach Kelsh. They helped me not just because I was a decent player with potential but because they actually cared. Both were aware of my home situation, and both of them went way above and beyond to keep me on the straight and narrow.

They devised a system to keep me attending class. It was simple. I had to have an attendance sheet signed by each of my teachers every day and then turn it in at the end of each school day. If I missed a class, I was off the team. This worked really well until basketball season ended. Once we were done, I could have cared less if I went or not.

School was two things to me, sports and girls. For some reason, I had no problem talking to girls. Communication was something I think I largely inherited from both of my parents as both could communicate really well. My Mother can speak well on almost any topic, even though she left school at a young age. She was a voracious reader, a trait that was passed on to me. Way before the internet was around, she bought us sets of children's and adult encyclopedias. Every day when I ate any meal other than supper, I read as I ate.

By the age of 15, I was barely passing my subjects. The exceptions being art (I had a natural ability to draw), English, and of course Phys Ed. Everything else was just a means to play basketball. I had made the Varsity Squad but was suspended off and on due to attendance issues. I didn't get tons of playing time as I was playing against 16-18-

year-olds but was happy to be on the team. On one occasion late in the game, Coach Kelsh called my name, "Todd, sub in for Danny!"

"Here we go!" was my thought, and I checked into the game. I was only in for a few minutes, but the blinders were in place. I did everything I was supposed to do. I didn't let the man I was guarding score. I was never out of position. I even got open twice, and both times that I shot, I scored!

When Coach Kelsh pulled me back out, he was really pleased! I could hear it in his voice, "WAY TO GO TODD! GREAT JOB OUT THERE!" I was elated. We won the game, and I was happy to have contributed more than just yelling from the bench for a change. I walked home in a really good mood.

The next day, my alarm went off. Waking up, I felt terrible. It's hard to explain. I should have felt great, on top of the world. For some reason, I just could not get out of bed. The thought of facing everyone at school was too much, and I simply hid. I ignored my Mother's calls to go to school until she left for work. I stayed in bed. Around 10:00 am, the phone started to ring. I knew who it was; it was Coach. I let it ring. He called repeatedly. Over and over. Finally, the ringing stopped. Fifteen minutes later, the doorbell rang. I crawled to the window and peaked outside. Sure enough, there was Coach Kelsh's car. "Ohhhhhh nooooo," I thought, and my mind began to race. What the hell was I supposed to do now? I sure wasn't going to answer the door. Was he going to beat the crap out of me? I hid until the doorbell stopped ringing, and he drove away. Getting dressed as fast as I could, my only recourse was to get to school. I made it in time for all of my afternoon classes.

During the last class, Coach had me paged to his office. When I got there, he simply motioned for me to sit, and like an obedient dog, I did. "Where were you this morning? You were not in class." I said nothing, just stared at the floor. "I came by your house Todd, why didn't you answer the door?" I could hear the frustration in his voice.

I fumbled some lie about just being out.

He pressed on, "I don't get it, Todd, you had a great game last night. So much potential! You are throwing it away. Why? All you have to do is go to class." I tried to explain but could not find the words. I was close to tears, close to losing it. How do you explain to someone that you look up to that you feel like a loser most of the time? I know now that I simply did not feel I deserved success; I did not know how to process good. It was and still is my nature to self-sabotage (knowing is half the battle). Mr. Kelsh was a good teacher, coach, and most importantly, he was a good man. He could see I was going to snap. He put his hand on my shoulder and said, "I'm not suspending you. Don't do it again, ok?" I couldn't look at him. I simply nodded. "Practice tomorrow after school, go home." I did my best to go to class after that, but I still had bouts of these dark times that I didn't know how to handle. I was crashing and heading towards a wall at a breakneck speed.

My Mom was running out of options with me. I didn't listen to her as I physically did not fear her. Also, I truly believed she hated me, so why listen? I was existing and not much else. I was only feeling alive when playing ball or boxing.

Mom had been through hell with Linda. She had been ostracized at school for pissing off some stupid little snot of a girl named Erminia when she was in grade eight. This little shit and her friends made Linda's life hell, all over some pants she wore to a dance. That's all it took. Linda was and is very tough. If you cross her, she will not forget it. Linda became one of the "tough kids," and it was best to stay out of her way.

Between dealing with Linda and then me, Mom was exhausted, and the stress was taking a toll on her mentally and physically. She had no backup and zero help from anyone.

I was pushing her to the limit. She was stressed, and rightfully so. Does that excuse the verbal and physical abuse over the years? She had been dealing with extreme circumstances for a long time, and she was human after all. She was running on fumes. She went to see her doctor and told him everything that was going on with me and how she didn't think she could handle me anymore.

I remember a few weeks earlier, there had been a fight between us. We were screaming at each other, not sure over what. She wound up to hit me. I caught the blow by her wrist and said, "You will never hit me again!" What an awful expression she had at that moment. She looked afraid and lost. I wish I would have let her hit me instead of seeing how she looked at me just then.

The doctor asked how old I was, and she said, "Sixteen." He offered her a solution.

That evening when I came home from school, my Mom called me from her bedroom. I peeked in.

"I want to talk to you, Todd."

The tone in her voice was unlike any I heard before. It was eerily cold. I remember getting a sick feeling to my stomach.

She continued, "You can't live here anymore. You are sixteen now, and that means legally, I do not have to look after you. You have to leave."

Stunned best describes my feeling upon hearing those words, and then I felt a new low. I figured I had been right all along. My own Mother hated me.

She then asked me the worst question I have ever been asked in my life, "I'm going to give you some money. How much do you think you are worth?" It took me a lot of years to forgive her for that moment. I am not even sure she knows why she asked it. Why was she being so cruel?

Maybe it was easier for her that way. She was making her only son leave after all because her doctor said it was a good idea. I told her I didn't want to leave. I was fighting back the anger and tears all at once.

"When do I have to go?"

"Tonight." was her reply.

She asked again, "How much do you think you are worth?" It hurt worse hearing it the second time.

My answer gives a pretty good indication of where I was emotionally and what I thought of myself.

Quietly I mumbled, "I don't know, fifty bucks?" I remember thinking she will never give me fifty bucks.

Her response shocked me, "I am giving you two thousand dollars. It is everything I was saving to help you with college one day. So now pack your bag and go. Make the best of it."

No "goodbye" or "I wish you luck." Certainly, no "I love you."

I went into my room, cheque in hand, and quietly packed my gym bag with as much of my stuff as I could. I walked out the front door with absolutely no plan or idea what to do.

"Now what?" was my first thought.

Then there was that spark, that quiet voice in my head, "Shoulder down Todd, take the space, drive hard to the hoop!"

Coach K's words. Always there. I was developing a skill. This was the biggest test of that skill. That skill was to survive. To adapt and survive. After all, in my head, I was worth fifty bucks!!!

CHAPTER 11

Twenty Thousand Pizzas

Sixteen years old, on my own. Up until the day my Mom kicked me out, I had probably never had more than fifty bucks to my name. Now here I was, standing on the front steps of the house I grew up in, a gym bag packed with everything I could fit into it and a cheque from my Mother for two thousand bucks.

"Now what?" I thought to myself. Luckily, survival mode set in. I did not have time to feel sorry for myself—no time to process what just happened. I needed to find a place to sleep. It was late fall, and Winnipeg is one cold place come fall and winter. Time to see what I was made of. Shoulder down.

First things first: cash the cheque.

I walked to the bank that my Mom dealt with and made it there before they closed. I had never cashed a cheque before. I looked over the tellers' faces, scanning each one carefully, hoping to find someone that looked kind.

There was no one in the bank at the time. My eyes locked onto the face of an attractive middle-aged woman; today, she would be referred to as a "cougar."

I smiled at her, she smiled back and asked, "May I help you?"

This was just one of many times that being able to communicate well, especially with women, would work in my favour.

I carefully explained my situation, changing some of the details about my Mom and the nature of our relationship. I made it look like Mom and I came to an agreement together so that she could better look after my younger sister.

After all, I was a young man and could look after myself.

She explained that normally they put a hold on cheques, but under the circumstances, she would see what she could do as long as I had proper identification. She disappeared into one of the offices, cheque in hand.

After a few minutes, she returned with a big smile and proceeded to count out twenty, crisp $100 dollar bills. She handed them to me and wished me the best of luck.

As I left, I thought to myself, "Okay, moron, you have some money. What's the next step?"

You couldn't say I had a large circle of friends because I did not.

As a whole, I did not trust many people. I could converse with almost anyone, but trusting someone was a whole different ball game. There were three fellows I considered close friends. It was largely because of my friends that I did not spend much time outdoors after being kicked out.

Rob Kliewer.

I had known Rob since the age of about seven. Rob came from a hard-working blue-collar German/Mennonite family with staunch Christian beliefs. We became friends simply because our older sisters were friends. Linda had asked me if I knew Rob. I didn't because even though we were the same age, he was in the grade younger than me.

My birth date made me one of those odd kids that could have been in either grade. My Mom started me early, not because I was advanced, more because I think she wanted me out of her hair! I still remember seeking Rob out in our playground at school.

In our first conversation, we spoke of our older sisters. He confessed to beating up his older sister Anita which impressed me immediately! As the thought of beating up Linda was unthinkable, she could kick the ass of most of the boys in her grade. From that day forward, we were fast friends.

Trevor King.

Trev moved into our Elmwood group when we were 12 or 13 years old. We had all known each other since kindergarten; there was a pecking order. We all knew who to mess with, whose ass you could kick, and who could kick yours! He was new blood. An unknown. It had been decided that we had to find out what this new kid was made of. He was pretty quiet, not athletic, and he seemed quite awkward. I had started boxing by this time, so our little group elected me to see what Trevor could do. What transpired is not a moment I am proud of. We were all hanging around, and as we had agreed, I tried to pick a fight with Trevor. He would have none of it. He wasn't a coward, not in the least. He was just not a fighter. To be honest with you, Trevor was smarter than all of us put together in many ways, and I don't think he saw any point in it.

Nonetheless, I persisted. When he would not take the bait, I started smacking him around—open-handed shots, to the shoulders, body, and arms. I started hitting him harder, trying to get him to engage. He did not. He stoically stood there and took it. He would not compromise what he believed in because of this nonsense.

Had he fought back, I would have destroyed him as I had the advantage of not only boxing but growing up in our group, we had spent years kicking the crap out of each other. I landed a hard shot to his shoulder, "COME ON!" I shouted.

Then I saw something I will never forget. Trevor's eyes were starting to water. "Aw hell," I thought, "don't cry, man!" Had Trevor cried, he would have been tormented from that day forward. I felt like the biggest ass in the world, no better than Jeff, who tormented me in the boxing ring every chance he got.

I made a decision. The exact words I used escape me, but in a nutshell, I told him to go home. Trev left. Once gone, I tried to turn things around.

"Wow, guys!" I said, "Trevor's all right. He didn't back down at all!" Which was, after all, the truth. He had guts, just no fighting ability. He was and is, to this day, one of the best people I know. He was accepted into our group, and as far as I know, nobody ever picked on him.

Not long after, I discovered we shared a love of 50's rock and roll as well as blues music. We spent many hours walking around our little neighborhood, singing our lungs out and getting into ridiculous situations while trying to impress girls!

Cory Stockwell.

Cory was a year younger than me and lived with his grandmother, whom he referred to as "Bunhead" or simply, "Bun." When I asked why he called her Bunhead, he explained it was because when he was very little, it was in reference to how she wore her hair in a bun. The name stuck, and Bunhead it was ever since.

Like myself, he was a basketball fanatic which made it easy for us to become good friends as we both would outlast everyone else in the gym, playing ball until they kicked us out. Cory was a year and a half younger than me (which he brought up EVERY time I beat him in a game of one-on-one.) He was adamant that that was the only reason I beat him.

To be honest, I was naturally quicker than Cory and could out-jump him. However, as sound as I was fundamentally, Cory could shoot the lights out and worked so hard on his entire game that he became a much more complete player than I, and he eventually became the best player on the team.

We had many great battles, and he would lose his mind if I beat him at any of the games we played, which was half the fun! My absolute favorite thing to do to him was immediately after one-on-one games. I would invariably beat him, which of course, would drive him nuts.

Then he would ask, "Did you have to try hard to win?'

My reply was always the same, "Not really."

Then he would get really mad. Twenty seconds later, he would look at me and say, "Okay, let's go again!"

Truth be told, it took everything I had to beat him. He was great. In a game, he was way better than me. I just was a very good one-on-one player. Shoulder down had served me well!

After cashing the cheque, the only place I could think of to go was Rob's house. His parents always made me feel welcome. They had fed me many meals over the years and even brought me out to their cabin located at Wanasing Beach when I was 11 years old. Strict and Christian, they worked very hard to put Rob and Anita through a private Christian school. Their house was very different than mine. There was no fear there. I loved those people.

Rob was home, and we went into his room. I said, "Close your eyes. I have to show you something!" He closed his eyes, and I fanned out all the bills. "Open," I said.

When Rob opened his eyes, he had a look of shock on his face that I can still picture today. "What d-did you do?" he quietly stammered, which I thought was hilarious, and burst out laughing.

I explained the whole thing to him as he listened. He didn't seem shocked, though, as he knew my home life all too well.

As we often did, we started making light of the situation. For me, it was a coping mechanism. Rob and I could crack each other up to the point of laughing so hard it hurt. On occasion, if I had ten bucks, I would often buy us pizza, and we would hang at his place and eat it together. So, when he asked what I was going to do with the two thousand bucks, I thought for a second and answered slowly, "I am going to buy TWENTY THOUSAND PIZZAS!!!" Of course, we thought that was the funniest thing in the world! We could not stop laughing.

Then it dawned on us how bad my math was, and that caused us to break out laughing all over again! Twenty thousand pizzas sounded way better, though, so we stuck with that! We then went out and bought a pizza, stayed up late talking about girls and nonsense. His parents let me crash there for the night. I had survived day one.

CHAPTER 12

Thank God for Pancakes!

They say you can never go home again. Perhaps there is some truth to that statement. Even though my home life had been less than ideal, it was still home. Perhaps it's normal as an adult to look back and remember the safety of being a child. Whatever level of safety one might have had. I had experienced some pretty awful things as a child, seen terrible things. There were also times of happiness. My Mom was great at taking care of us at Christmas. There were certain meals my Mother cooked that I would give anything to have again! I had my own room and didn't have to worry about where my next meal was coming from.

It didn't hit me right away, but there was a certain loneliness that started to set in shortly after my Mom had kicked me out. Was my family messed up? Yes, it was, but isn't that true of every family to some degree?

Realizing that you are not welcome in your family home hurts profoundly. Wasn't your family supposed to be there for you? My self-esteem was not great at the best of times, and now it was at an all-time low.

I was bouncing around, sleeping at different friend's houses. Outside at times. I was showering at school and washing my clothes wherever and whenever I could—living off of peanut butter sandwiches. It was weird and unnerving.

Word travels fast, and having your peers know your parents kicked you out made you pretty vulnerable. I was on edge and in a bad place. I had asked my friends if I could maybe stay with them, that's a lot to ask of one's parents, and of course, the answer was always no. I tried to continue with school and sports, seeking some sort of stability. I was losing weight and not eating well.

I discovered what real hunger felt like. I was still playing basketball, but I let boxing go as there was no way I could do both living off of minimal food. Not to mention basketball was my first love and my preferred sport. It was becoming increasingly hard mentally as well as physically.

Once during practice, I got into it with one of my teammates—Mike Reid, who was very quick-witted and funny as hell.

I can't remember what we were fighting about, but I do remember one thing. A remark he made that crushed me. He yelled, "At least for my birthday, my parents didn't give me luggage!"

Everyone laughed hard at that one. I didn't laugh. It hurt. Basketball and classes were becoming less and less important. I didn't need this. It felt like I was slipping away.

It was my friend Rob's parents that saved me, really. I had spent many nights sleeping at their house. Mrs. Kliewer fed me many a meal. They never made me feel bad about my situation. They never preached at me either, despite their Christian beliefs. They lived it. They were not perfect by any stretch but simply put, they were good people.

I had been to church with them many times, and to be honest, I never felt welcome. They went to a large, mostly Mennonite/German church. A lot of the congregation was well off. They stuck together. If you did not have a German/Mennonite last name, you definitely felt like an outsider. These people did not know my parents or me. They really did not know how to categorize me. However, the Kliewer family never made me feel that way.

One memory that stuck out was one of Rob's Dad, Bruno. I remember that every time I slept there, in the morning, I would see Bruno sitting quietly by himself at the kitchen table reading his bible. No one around. Just him and the word of God. I thought that was a fine example of a good, humble Christian man. Not reading to show what a good Christian he was. It was how he started his day, every day. Witnessing that gave me a sense of peace.

Mrs. Kliewer worked in the kitchen of the Mennonite College that was next to the private school that Rob attended. She took it upon herself to help me find a place to live. I had no idea she was doing this. It was an amazing thing, really. She was very well-liked at the college as she just was a Mom to everyone. How could you not like her? She often took the time to chat with the students and became aware of two brothers Lloyd and Gerald Klassen, who were renting a side-by-side house a street over from the college with one other roommate, Merv

Voth. She asked them if they would consider another roommate, me! She told them of my situation, and they agreed to meet with me.

I was pretty nervous as I walked up the sidewalk of the dilapidated side-by-side. I had no idea what to expect. Mrs. Kliewer had given me the basics. That was it. Just that there were these three Christian students sharing a place and that they would consider letting me stay there.

"Here goes nothing!" I thought as I knocked on the door. "Better than sleeping outside" was my next realization.

The door opened, standing in front of me was a very attractive girl in her early 20's. I stood there with my mouth open and saying nothing, like an idiot.

"You must be Todd. Come on in"

I stepped inside and was immediately greeted by a young man in glasses, athletically built with a voice that sounded a tiny bit like Kermit, the frog, at times. "I'm Gerald, and this is my girlfriend Eileen. Welcome here!"

He sounded very genuine. The interior of the side-by-side was actually very homey. It felt warm and safe. I hadn't felt safe for some time. That feeling was very welcome. They invited me to sit down and asked me to tell my story. To the best of my ability, I did just that.

To my surprise, Gerald told me that it would be just fine if I moved in as long as I was ok with sleeping on a sofa and having what should have been the dining room as my bedroom! Ok? It was beyond ok with me! Big improvement over begging friends to ask their parents if I could sleepover, or worse yet, sleeping outside!

I settled in. My share of the rent was $50.00. Cheap even in those days as the total rent for the place was $200.00 per month, plus utilities. I had not used very much of the money Mom had given me, so for the first time, I felt a bit of peace of mind. It wasn't that I didn't miss home. I did. Especially on weekends when my roommates went back home, and I found myself all alone.

However, Gerald, Lloyd, and Merv all did their best to make me feel at home with them. They all played basketball. Merv was playing for the University of Winnipeg, which of course, was very impressive to me. He was six foot six inches tall, and for a basketball player, quite muscular and strong. When Merv was around, he took the time to play ball with me, which I loved, especially because he didn't go easy on me. If he could block every shot I took, he would. This, to me, was great because it taught me how to play against guys much bigger and stronger than me. Made me a better player. It made me tougher. It was a challenge, so of course, there was a huge appeal in that!

All three of the guys were Christian. Lloyd was the coolest of the three in a very hippy Christian way. He sported a long beard and hair, which was not common in the '80s. Although he didn't look it, he was a deceptively quick and gifted basketball player. The odd thing is that he didn't seem to run; he glided. It looked slow because it was so smooth. It was always fun to watch the bewildered look of the face of whoever was guarding him, as time and time again, he would blow by his opponent like they were standing still. He also had a dry sense of humour. I enjoyed hanging out with Lloyd because he was so cool, albeit on his own terms! He dressed how he wanted to, listened to strange music, had his belief system, and really didn't seem to care what anyone thought about any of it! It was a different type of strength that I had not encountered before.

Gerald was quieter than Lloyd in some ways, much more conservative-looking. He had an infectious laugh and was always there to listen to me if I needed a sounding board. His girlfriend Eileen was often at our little place, and she was not only very pretty but unbelievably sweet and kind. Very genuine. I came to view her as a sister and was very fond of both of them.

Gerald also joined in our pick-up basketball games. He was the type of player that could get on these shooting streaks where he would not miss. If he was on fire, he hit everything!

On the occasions he was not hitting, it was the complete opposite. He would hit nothing! Most players would stop shooting if they were cold, not Gerald. Hot or cold, Gerald shot every chance he got! The bad thing was, if he was cold, he would get very upset, and he did not hide it. In some ways, he was the total opposite of his brother Lloyd. I do not ever remember seeing Lloyd ever get upset by anything!

Big Merv. As big as he is, Merv is one of the kindest and most gentle people I have ever met. He was and is a Christian in every sense of the word. He tried his very best to influence me in a positive way. If he was around, he would make sure that I didn't cut class. In fact, one day, I had decided to sleep in despite his efforts to wake me up for school. All of a sudden, I could feel little drops of water hitting my forehead—drip, drip, drip. I woke up to see Merv standing over me with a bucket of water poised over my head as Merv quietly said, "Time to wake uuuuuup!" He had a huge smile on his face, and I knew without a doubt that he would take great pleasure in dumping the whole bucket on me to teach me a lesson! I was up immediately! One of my favorite memories of Merv was when we tried to play a practical joke on him. We were always playing jokes on each other, and in some ways, I felt much more like a college kid than a high school senior as I spent so much time with these guys and their friends. I always looked older than my age as a teen, I think due to my dark hair and looks, so I was largely accepted as one of them. On this one occasion, Merv was taking a bath. The house had no shower, just an old-fashioned claw-foot bathtub that was huge and deep! Lloyd and I got it into our heads that it might be funny to take the cat (aptly named Kitty) that lived in the house and throw it in the tub with Merv. We had visions of the cat freaking out and scratching the hell out of poor Merv! We thought this would be hilarious! So, Lloyd and I grab Kitty and slowly make our way upstairs towards the bathroom. The lock didn't work properly, so no problem there. My job was to open the door as Lloyd threw the poor cat at unsuspecting Merv! Lloyd whispered, "On the count of three, one, two, THREE!" I swung the door open, and Lloyd hurled poor Kitty at Merv. Never missing a beat, he caught Kitty as he hit the water and proceeded to not only calm Kitty down, he went on to give Kitty a bath as Lloyd and I stood there, our mouths hanging open in disbelief as Merv calmly dealt with Kitty. In a nutshell, that sums up Merv.

No matter what challenges life threw at him, Merv would not only deal with it, he would do so gladly. In his eyes, he was simply serving the Lord. He taught by example, by his actions. To this day, this is how Merv operates. He had a profound effect on me.

Over time, I started to feel more like a college student than a high school senior. One memory that really stands out occurred after we had finished a game of pick-up basketball at the High School gym that was connected to the Bible College. I was talking with Lloyd, and a very pretty brunette from the college approached us and started a conversation with me.

I was beyond thrilled. She was at least 20 years old, pretty, and well-spoken. We talked for several minutes as Lloyd watched with a bemused look on his face.

We were just at the point where I was about to ask for her number when Lloyd interjected, "You do know that Todd doesn't go to the college. He's still in high school."

With that, she quickly excused herself and walked away at a brisk pace.

I looked at Lloyd in disbelief. "WHY?" I sputtered.

Lloyd burst out laughing, "She would have found out anyway!"

We both ended up laughing pretty hard even though I wanted to kill him. He went on to explain that many young Christian women and men go to bible college with the hopes of meeting a husband or wife there. That's why Bible College was jokingly referred to as "Bridal College."

It made sense, really. You had all these young college kids, hormones raging. Yet, they are supposed to refrain from sex. Easy solution, get married!

To this day, I think a lot of those young marriages were more a result of out-of-control hormones than love. Let's face it; it's pretty easy to convince yourself you are in love when you are making out all the time, with no sex and all the great feelings that come with new, young relationships!

At the age of 16 – 20 years old, I was pretty sure I was in "love" with every girl that I dated or made out with. Realistically, I just wanted sex. My adolescent brain did not know the difference, and I certainly made a fool out of myself chasing girls. I had zero fear of asking girls out and never took it personally if they said no.

At a young age, I had realized that you are not going to be every girl's ideal, just as every girl may not be mine. If a girl said no when I asked her out, I simply said, "Thanks anyway," and went about my business. Having that kind of confidence going in was a huge advantage, and I found I was getting a lot more yes's than rejections.

The problem was, I had no clue at all how to be relaxed or be myself with any girl once in a relationship. The scars from growing up always came into play, and I was a wreck. As a result, most girlfriends stuck around for a month or so until one of us realized that we were not "meant to be."

My roommates tried their best to be positive influences on me. Merv even got me a job at the Bible Camp he worked at every summer. This morphed into me moving to a small town with a Christian Mennonite family that wanted to "help" me. It was a complete disaster.

I had learned to be somewhat of a chameleon as a survival skill over the years. Having a strong ability to communicate helped me to fit in with many types of social groups. I did my best to fit into their very regimented Christian household. Which I was able to do. It wouldn't last long. First of all, I have never done well with anyone telling me what to do. Second, I had already lived on my own. Third, it was a smaller, mostly German/Mennonite community. I stood out like a sore thumb with my dark hair and French last name. The experiment quickly failed, and I found myself back in Winnipeg in short order.

My Mom agreed to let me move back home. This would also prove to be a disaster. After being on my own, doing my own thing, not to mention I still carried a ton of resentment from being kicked out the first time. There was no way I could handle living at home any longer.

Before long, I found myself back with the boys in the side-by-side. It was not ideal, but still way better than home or the street. I had long ago gone through the money my Mom had given me to start out. I was still trying to go to school, mostly to play sports at this point.

I was working odd jobs here and there and barely getting by. Some days I did not eat much, if at all. Luckily Merv's Mom intervened to a degree. She pre-mixed a huge batch of pancake mix. It was literally a huge tub of the stuff. Merv shared it with the household. It was simple; you added water and cooked it in a pan. If not for that mix. I would have gone hungry many more days than I did. Some days it was quite literally pancakes for breakfast, lunch, and dinner. I remember thinking on more than one occasion, "Thank God for pancakes."

CHAPTER 13

Education of a Wannabe

It was becoming increasingly clear to me that Graduating from High School was not going to happen for me. I was 18 years old, already missing my grad year had I graduated on time. I was simply existing, going through the motions. Only going to classes I liked and playing sports. Direction in my life was needed in a big way, and I was lost as to what to do or what to pursue.

It has been said that everything happens for a reason, so perhaps it was inevitable that I would gravitate to bodybuilding. It had been many years since Jack LaLanne had inspired me to start exercising and pushing myself. I knew deep down that one day, and once high school sports were finished that I would begin my quest for a strong and muscular physique. The muscle magazines had always intrigued me. The bodybuilders looked like living art. Of course, they were big and strong, which also was something I greatly admired. However, the beauty and artistry of it appealed to me even more.

The impetus, or inspiration, that pushed me into the gym happened quite by chance. The volleyball season was winding down, and I knew this was the last high school sport I was going to participate in and also knew that I would not graduate or return to school the next year. It didn't seem important at the time, and I did not want to be 19 and still in high school. We had one more game to play, and our season was done. On this particular weekend, I was crashing at my friend Scott Samson's place. He lived with his Mom, a single parent, and she was not often at home from what I could see. We were just talking, hanging out, when I noticed a paperback book sitting on a table. On the cover was a very muscular individual. I picked it up. The title read, "Arnold, Education of a Bodybuilder." On the cover was a picture of none other than Arnold Schwarzenegger. He was hitting a bicep pose, and I stared in disbelief that anyone could have such a huge arm. Not only that, but the rest of his body looked perfect, almost mythical. I immediately asked Scott if I could borrow the book.

It was Arnold's first autobiography. He explained how he had first seen a Muscle Magazine with Mr. Universe Reg Park on the cover and how he immediately knew he wanted to be like him. Park had starred in many Hercules and sword and sandal films as a result of having this heroic physique. Arnold grew up in Thal, a tiny village in Austria. Bodybuilding was virtually unknown there, and Arnold being Arnold, told anyone who would listen that he was going to become the best-built man in the world. After that, he explained he would move to America and become a movie star. He was 15 at the time, and everyone thought he was crazy, telling him it was impossible. His parents did not understand his ambitions. They, like everyone else, did their best to dissuade him from what seemed to be an impossible dream. Of course, we all knew what happened. Arnold made good on his word, becoming, in fact, not only the best-built man in the world but so revered in bodybuilding that even today, many experts believe he was the best bodybuilder of all time! Then, of course, he became the highest-paid movie star in the world for many years and then, of course later, even more incredulous, the Governor of the State of California!

His body more than impressed me. I loved the idea of sculpting one's body to shape it into living art—art that was strong and beautiful. Also, there was the challenge of it. In the 80's you just did not see very many bodybuilders walking around. In being one, you were pretty much guaranteed to stand out and be unique. I already felt different or like an outsider for years, but not for the right reasons. Now I wanted to be different all over again and do something that most would not or could not do!

As much as Arnold's body impressed me (still does), it was his WILL, his drive, and goal setting that really spoke to me. I could really identify with people saying, "You can't do it. It's impossible." That drove me more than anything. When I was told no, I heard yes! Arnold's whole life epitomized that very philosophy!

I read the book that night—cover to cover. There was a section on training, complete with routines and nutritional guidelines. There were many pictures of Arnold, of course. The one that stood out the most to me was taken when he was only 19. He had been training for four years and already weighed about 250 – 260lbs. He was massive but with fantastic proportions. The backdrop in the photo was the Swiss Alps. He looked amazing and strong. I could not get over the fact that he was only 19 years old with this type of physique! I knew nothing of genetics or steroids at that time. To me, seeing was believing. So, if this Arnold Schwarzenschnitzel (as Arnold often jokingly refers to himself as) could do it, if Reg Park could do it, well then, of course, I could do it!

"Scott!" I exclaimed, "We HAVE to do this! Once volleyball is over, we have to train for bodybuilding! Arnold says it's good to train with a buddy for motivation, so let's train together! What do you think?"

Scott agreed. Hell, his last name was Samson! It's like being named Thor or Hercules! Of course, he should lift weights! We agreed that the day after the last game that we would meet after school in the school weight room.

I wrote out one of Arnold's "intermediate" workout plans for us to follow. In my mind, being an athlete meant that the beginner routines were beneath me. Of course, I could handle more, or so I thought.

The day after our last game, I couldn't wait for classes to end so I could take the first step towards becoming like Arnold. I waited for 20 minutes for Scott. He never showed. "Screw it!" I thought. "I'm done waiting!"

Thus, I took my first workout. Chest and back were the body parts being worked on. I did every set and every rep that Arnold's workout called for. The feeling of the "pump" was amazing. Blood rushes into the muscle being worked, making it feel swollen and larger. I quickly fell in love with that feeling.

Morning. I had been sore in my life before, from basketball, boxing, running. I knew what sore felt like. It didn't bother me. THIS, however, was like nothing I had ever felt in my life. With every movement, I felt shooting pain in what seemed to be every muscle in my upper body! I could barely wash my hair! Most normal or, let's say, sane people, do not associate that type of pain with anything positive. To me, this was great! I figured that I must have done something right to be this sore. Soreness equals growth, progress. It made total sense in my mind. I had surmised that if I wasn't sore, it would mean I babied myself, that I did not work hard enough to induce growth.

Scott never did get into training, despite his last name. I think when he saw how much pain I was in the next day that perhaps bodybuilding was for crazy people!

My first workouts took place in our high school gym after school Monday – Friday. Arnold's plans also called for a workout on Saturday, so I was training six days per week, close to two hours each day.

With the school being closed on Saturdays, I began going to the North End YMCA. The North End of Winnipeg was a short walk from my neighborhood and has long been one of the toughest areas in the city. That did not deter me one bit. In fact, once the school year finished, I began training there six days per week.

The gym itself was small and very hot and humid in the summer as it was adjacent to the indoor pool in the basement. Training there, working up a sweat was not a problem. I took my workouts very seriously, and the tunnel vision I had used to focus on improving my basketball skills came in very handy. I took it so seriously that I once knocked one of my first training partners to the ground for fooling around during our workout. He was training for fun. I had a goal and got very mad that his goofing off was getting in the way. We started exchanging heated words as I challenged his manhood, work ethic and asked him why he was so gutless. He told me where I could go, and I punched him in the chest as hard as I could. After he got up, I realized what I had done and began to apologize, but it was too late, and that was the end of his training with me. I don't remember his name. He was just one of the guys that were training at the Y. I became completely obsessed with training and changing my body.

The first six to twelve months of training can be the most amazing time for muscular growth. If a person has some decent genetics, trains hard and consistently as well as feeding the body adequately the gains can be outstanding!

Everything you do basically shocks the muscle into growth as the stimulus of lifting weights is so new to the body. The body simply adapts to this new workload by growing both in muscular size and strength.

Sadly, these gains do not continue at this pace for long, and, over time, I learned that you had to constantly shock the muscles into growth with different training methods: heavy weights and low reps, or lighter weight and high reps. Forced reps, drop sets, compound free-weight movements vs. machines, cables, and isolation work. Different training splits.

Really the variations were endless. It is tough, grueling work. The body will get used to different workouts quite quickly, and it easy to get into a routine and stick to the exercises that we like the best. However, once in a comfort zone, the growth stops as the muscle has no reason to grow as it becomes accustomed to the current workload.

For the next several months, the North End Y became my home away from home. I became friends with the regulars that trained at the same time of day that I did. Many of us were anxious to become as big and strong as we could. We pushed each other, spotted each other on heavy lifts, and exchanged bits of training info that we picked up from various bodybuilding magazines and books on the subject. It was small and often crowded and definitely smelled like a gym.

Most of us knew very little about training, and more often than not, it was the blind leading the blind. Then there was Adolph, by far the biggest guy in our gym and also the scariest. At about five foot ten and around 240 solid lbs, he definitely cast a large shadow.

Adolph was of aboriginal descent, covered in tattoos, and was menacingly quiet. In the '80s, tattoos were not as common as today. Back then, they were the domain of members of the military, biker gangs, convicts and ex-cons, and serious badass individuals as a rule.

He had recently been released from prison for an assault charge. Apparently, he threw some unlucky fellow through a second-story plate glass window. As intimidating as he was, I studied him. I watched him train. He would bench press 315lbs with ease. I had only seen pictures of guys doing that in the magazines. Up close, it was very impressive.

The iron plates would clang and sing with each rep, and when he completed a set (never having anyone spot him), he would rack the weight himself. Gradually I started talking to Adolph. As far as I knew, no one else dared to. It started with a head nod. Then graduated to saying, "Hi."

Eventually, I started asking questions about his training. He patiently answered each one. This became a pattern for me, find the biggest or strongest fellow in the gym and gather as much information as I could by observing and respectfully asking questions in between sets or at the end of workouts.

My body was changing. Growth was occurring. I still remember the first time someone noticed that I was growing. It was Mark Koop that first said something. He went to the same private school that Rob went to. Like myself, he was an avid basketball player, and I knew him from many pick-up games at his school and also at his house on his driveway court.

We were all hanging out at the Kliewer's house, and I was wearing a t-shirt. Mark was staring at my arms and asked, "Todd, have you been working out? Lifting weights or something? Cause your arms look bigger."

It was amazing to hear this! Someone could tell I was growing! It was really happening, just like Arnold had said! The education of a wannabe had begun!

CHAPTER 14

Olympik Gym

Since my less than stellar high school career had come to an end, it was now time to get on with life and find a full-time job to support myself and my bodybuilding lifestyle, which at this point meant vast quantities of food! You need fuel to grow, and that meant eating 6-7 calorie-dense meals per day. I was, in fact, growing and getting stronger, but in my mind, it was not happening nearly fast enough. Every article about gaining mass that I read said that you must eat to grow. And eat I did!

I had found a full-time job at a sports equipment store selling sneakers. It was boring, and I was amazed at how much the markup was on a pair of athletic shoes of any kind. My boss was a small, nebbish, bald-headed man that looked more weasel than man and had a personality to match. He was constantly chewing his nails and looking like he wanted to be anywhere but at the store dealing with customers.

He hated me and was constantly on me to put out as much effort into selling sneakers as I put into lifting weights. I, of course, found that to be hilarious. With as much patience as I could, I dealt with customers all day while dreaming of California, Muscle Beach, and the bodybuilding lifestyle.

Much of that was fiction created by Joe Weider to sell his Muscle Magazines, training courses, and, of course, his supplements. In my mind, it all looked like heaven: working out, playing in the ocean, and your pick of beautiful bikini-clad women!

One day when I was goofing off (something I did as much as I could), a very built man in his 20's came into the store. He was about five foot eight and impossibly thick. I quickly introduced myself and immediately turned the conversation into one about bodybuilding. I asked him where he trained.

His reply was "Olympik Gym."

I had never heard of it, and when I asked him where it was, he said, "Elmwood."

As it turned out, this little gem of a training dungeon quietly existed not five minutes from where I lived. I got the address and promised myself come hell or high water and I would find this gym the next day!

The following day, I could not get out of work fast enough. I got home, changed into my gym clothes, and set out. Finding the building where the gym was housed was easy. However, it was evident to me why I had never heard of it. It was in the back of a building that also was a storage facility for mattresses. The front of the building was a support facility for special needs children and adults.

Tucked in the back in between the two was a door with a small sign simply reading, "Olympik Gym." There were no windows, only an overhead door that would be opened when the weather permitted. This was no shiny commercial gym. I would later find out that it was owned by six guys that simply wanted a real gym to train in. It was not meant to be a commercial gym at all. They just wanted to make enough money to keep the lights on!

When I walked in, I felt like I stepped into a time machine. All free weights, nothing chrome, no cardio machines, save one dilapidated stationary bike that looked like the kind you found in your high school weight room. The walls were cinder block. The back wall had a huge painting of "Ollie," the gym's muscular cartoon mascot. It was Olympik's version of the Gold's Gym guy. Ollie was grimacing as he curled a massive weight. I must have looked like a deer caught in someone's headlights as I stared with a dopey grin on my face.

My trance was broken when I heard a very loud voice call out, "Hey! You lost kid? You need sumthin?"

I feebly answered, "I want to join the gym."

His reply was simple and to the point, "$25.00 a month!"

Until this moment, I had not looked at the person talking to me. When I looked over at him, I was a bit taken aback. His name was Bruce Markham. A bulldog of a man in every sense of the word. At maybe 5 foot five inches tall, I had never seen someone that height with so much muscle. His body was thick all over, and he sported a close-cropped head of red hair with a red moustache that reminded me of an old-time strong man. He was a Canadian Champion in powerlifting, which he won competing without drugs of any kind, and made it all the way to the world championships on more than one occasion. He was one of Olympik's owners as well.

I handed Bruce my crumpled-up $25.00 and decided to train immediately. It would be legs that day which, of course, meant squats. To begin, I warmed up with the empty bar, which weighed 45lbs, and then slowly added weight to each set until I was at 225lbs, which at that time was a fair bit of weight for me.

As I was doing my set, I heard Bruce call out, "What the fuck are you doing?"

I kept doing reps, thinking to myself, "I wonder who he is talking to?"

Then he yelled it a second time.

"There is no way he is talking to me," I thought as I completed my set and racked the weight.

I turned around to see the human bulldog glaring at me, and he was now right behind me.

"I said, what the fuck are YOU doing?"

"Oh crap!" I thought, "He WAS talking to me!"

"I'm doing squats," I stammered.

"That is not how you squat. Get out of the way, and pay attention!" Bruce instructed.

Then without any warmup sets, Bruce shouldered the 225lbs and squatted deeper than anyone I had ever seen.

While in the bottom position, he explained, "This is how deep you should be going! The only thing you are working on by going halfway down is your ego!"

He performed several more reps so easily it looked like there was no weight on the bar. When it was my turn, he had me remove 90lbs of weight, leaving a mere 135lbs on the bar. He then patiently taught me how to squat properly. The difference was night and day! Performing deep squats or ass to the grass squats, as Bruce called them, was much harder than the half squats I had been doing.

He then asked if I knew how to deadlift. I did not. So that was next, deadlifts, and those hurt more than the squats! By the time he was done teaching me those, I was completely spent. TWO EXERCISES! That was it, and I had nothing left. Up until that point, I thought I was training hard. My education in bodybuilding and powerlifting was about to begin in earnest!!!

Finding a better facility in which to learn how to train would have been pretty tough to do in the 1980s in Winnipeg. Per square foot, you could not find a gym that produced anyone stronger than Olympik. There were, of course, bigger gyms around, but they often went the way of the ill-fated Dodo bird or often changed owners several times until finally shutting their doors for good.

We were a tight-knit group of lifters at Olympik. The gym itself was small, at best a little over 1000 square feet. Before long, I was offered a job there to run the gym during the day and clean the equipment and washrooms. That was heaven for me at that time in my life. The best time of the day was right around 5:00 pm. It was then that the regulars and heavy lifters trained. That little place would come alive with an energy that was sure to get anyone pumped up! It was a real man's gym.

There were women that trained there as well, more often than not, spouses or girlfriends of some of the guys. Any other women that ventured into our little cave were usually pretty serious about training and could definitely hold their own!

Olympik was not for the faint of heart. We all competed against each other, egged each other on, and there was no shortage of sarcasm! May God help you if you trained with bad form, did not train hard, or only trained the "bar muscles." Namely, chest and biceps.

There was minimal steroid use, and those that did partake in anabolic experimentation certainly kept it low-key, and it was not discussed as openly as it is in most gyms today. It was not unusual for new members that really did not understand our gym etiquette to quickly be vanquished from our little club. They were not asked to leave per se; they didn't have to be. Some of our regulars would simply mock them until they left. Survival of the fittest, and we looked after our own.

I was not spared the sarcasm, and I was taught many a lesson the hard way! For example, when I first started training there, I had fallen in love with the bench press. I was determined to have an impressive chest like Arnold's, and I really enjoyed the feeling of that particular lift.

I began to overtrain my chest, sometimes benching two or three times per week. I trained the rest of my body as well, but not with the same enthusiasm as my chest. The guys started to pick up on that, especially one heavyweight bodybuilder named Kevin Lunney and his training partner Trevor Wallace. Kevin was 6ft tall and resembled a

250lb muscular Tom Selleck. He was a REAL bodybuilder, and I looked up to him as it seemed he had muscles everywhere, not just bar muscles! Kevin also had a confidence that bordered on cockiness at times. He used his very dry sense of humour and observations to cut you down pretty damn quick if he felt you needed it.

In my life, I do not believe I have ever witnessed ANYONE that trained as hard as Kevin. He trained six days per week come hell or high water, and his workouts were extremely high volume using the heaviest weights possible with the proper form, I might add! These torture sessions lasted a MINIMUM of two hours each day.

His training partner, Trevor, was about five foot eight with one of the widest backs I had ever seen. It was massive—like block out the sun massive. He was strong as hell. He didn't just LOOK strong; he was the real deal. Trevor also shared Kevin's sense of humour and, in fact, was the funnier of the two. They snapped me out of doing too much bench pressing and overtraining my chest. As soon as I walked in the gym, I would be greeted by one of them saying, "Hey Todd, let me guess, chest day? Bench press?"

It was a small gym, and all of the regulars heard it, and it usually got a good laugh, even more so if I was actually training chest that day! It did not take too long for me to start giving the rest of my body parts equal attention and to give bench press a much-needed break. Was it mean? Not really. It was simply their way of saying, "If you are going to train here, train smart!" They just used sarcasm to hit their point home. If you were too thin-skinned for that, you would never last! Go to a "fitness centre" if you can't take the heat was the creed of our little dungeon!

Another time I had decided to try some "high-intensity training" that consisted of abbreviated workouts with minimal training days (only three per week), with minimal sets and maybe 40 minutes in the gym each session. No one at Olympik trained like that. Everyone lifted heavy with medium to high volume training. Some of the powerlifters trained four days per week, but they were lifting such heavy weights that training any more than four days would not be adequate recovery time.

The first day I tried out my "HIT" program, the workout took only about 35 minutes. When I was finished, I started getting ready to leave, and of course, Kevin and Trevor noticed. Kevin called out to me as I was heading out, "Where do you think you're going?"

As I started to reply that I was done, Trevor interjected, "Oh, I know that workout! That's the Jane Fonda 20-minute workout!" With that comment, all the regulars erupted with laughter, and I felt my face turn very red as I left with no comeback at all.

The next day was supposed to be a day off as the routine called for training on Monday, Wednesday, and Fridays only.

When I returned on Wednesday to train, Kevin spotted me entering and asked, "Where were you yesterday?"

I explained that on this program, you only train three days per week. That was met with a reply of, "Makes sense! If you want to look like Jane Fonda, you don't want to train too much!"

Again, loud laughter erupted from everyone, and that was the end of my HIT program. I couldn't help but laugh as well. Again, it was their way of saying, "Don't waste your time with that garbage! Train hard, get big and get strong!" These guys were like tough coaches and knew more about training than 95% of the people that call themselves "trainers" today! These lessons that were taught to me daily are something I could not put a price on!

I learned the art of sarcasm quickly and became an accepted member of that little brotherhood. Despite the put-downs and smart-ass comments, you could not find a more supportive group. If someone was attempting a big lift or a new personal best, it was not unusual for everyone to stop what they were doing to cheer on the lifter.

You would hear shouts of, "C'mon man, you got this! Light weight! Stay tight, remember to explode!!!" After the lift, everyone would be saying, "Right on! Great lift!" and patting the guy (or girl) on the back.

If you missed the lift, everyone would be just as supportive with great insights as to why the lift was missed. This was a group of very advanced lifters that could see that perhaps on your deadlift, you didn't drive hard enough through your hips. Or perhaps you got out of your groove on the bench press attempt. This was not something you could find in most commercial gyms.

I still remember the first time I benched two plates (225lbs). Two plates were very intimidating to me at the time! It meant that there would be two large 45lb plates on each side of the barbell. I had been stuck at 215lbs for weeks and could not get past my fear of that next level. That was a weight the "bigger" guys lifted.

At that point, in my mind, it was simply too much! On this particular day, I had performed my warmup sets and was about to do my usual 215lb bench press when I heard a familiar voice behind me, "Why don't you move up to two plates?"

I turned around. It was Danny Tarabulka. One of Olympik's owners. Danny stood about six feet tall and competitively lifted at a bodyweight of about 198lbs. Solidly built but not massive, he was amazingly powerful. Danny mainly trained with his wife Gwen, who was such a sweet lady and fit in very well with our little group. Dan was a very accomplished lifter setting many deadlift records. He was like a human crane! He would pull 500lb deadlifts like it was nothing for reps, and when he was going heavy would easily go over 600lbs. Everyone respected him a great deal, and he was a real positive influence on everyone in the gym.

"Dan, I don't think I can press 225lbs!" was my reply.

He shook his head, "That's your first problem. What you are thinking is holding you back. I have watched you press 215lbs for weeks now. It's a mental block. Trust me. You ARE strong enough, at least your body is. The key is believing it! Right now, the only thing stopping you is your negative thoughts! Today you are going to press 225lbs. I am going to help you. How many reps can you get with 215lbs?"

"On a good day, usually about eight." I answered.

"Ok, great! I am going to spot you, and I only want you to do four reps, ok? Very important, each rep, I want you to totally control the weight. Control the speed on the way down. Once that bar touches your chest, explode it up! Make it look easy. It's only four reps!"

With that, I chalked up my hands and got ready as Danny positioned himself behind the bench.

"Ok, Todd, I'm going to give you a lift-off. I will count off, one, two, three, and give the command, 'Lift.' When I say lift, we go! Focus, it's light weight, only four reps." I steadied myself under the bar as Danny counted off. The reps seemed easy. After all, I usually was pushing to get eight reps.

I racked the weight, and Danny and I loaded the barbell, so it now had two 45lb plates on each side. It was a mental block, all right. Looking at those two big 45lb plates on each side made me shudder.

At the time, it just looked HEAVY! I got back into position, and Danny started speaking to me in a quiet voice, "Ok, here we go. Focus. This isn't heavy. We are going to take it off the rack. Steady it and control the descent. You got this. Once the bar touches, you are going to rip it off your chest so hard it's going to go through the ceiling!"

Those words, spoken like that, put me into a zone. It was like everything fell away. I could see in my mind everything he described. The doubts vanished. "Shoulder down!" It was as if I could hear Coach K's voice as well.

Danny counted off, "One, two, three, LIFT!"

With that, we unracked the weight. I steadied it and smoothly brought it down to my chest. As soon as the bar touched, I immediately powered it up with such force it caught me by surprise! At the completion of the rep, Danny called for another rep and then a third! I racked the weight and sat up immediately with a stunned look on my face. It was then I heard the other gym members exclaiming, "Good lift! Way to go!" Everyone had stopped to watch and give their support.

Now it's not that a 225lb bench press is any big deal; it's not a great amount by any stretch. However, at that time, it was a big deal to me. The positive energy from the guys in the gym felt fantastic. I felt like I belonged and mattered, which was something that was foreign to me. It was amazing!

Maybe I did not realize it at the time, but I had begun to learn some very valuable lessons. Until that point, I had realized the importance of visualization when it came to training or athletics. The only reason I had not been able to press 225lbs before that day was that I BELIEVED I could not. Danny had painted a picture in my mind so clearly that any doubts I had about making that lift were gone before we even unracked the weight. Once the fear and doubt were removed, I not only was able to complete the lift, two additional reps became possible!

From that day forward, whenever I was attempting a big lift in bench, squat, or deadlift, I would have Danny spot me if he was in the gym. He was able to get in my head in such a way that I never missed a lift when he was spotting me. He would talk me through it so effectively it was like being hypnotized or in a trance. He would describe the lift, how it would feel, what to expect. By the time I attempted the lift, in my mind, I had already successfully completed it.

The actual lift was a matter of fact. Also, having always believed in role models and mentors, there was part of me that felt if I failed, on some level, I would be letting Danny down. There was no way I was going to let that happen.

To this day, I can still hear Danny's words whenever I am about to try a heavy lift, sometimes I speak them aloud, and it never fails to get me into the right mental space. Like anything, this is a skill that is honed through practice. I can't remember the last time I missed a lift. My best guess is about three years ago attempting a 495lb decline press. The next time I attempted it, I was successful, which was later that same month. Now, whenever I am coaching someone through a big lift, it is Danny's words that I speak to get the lifter into the right mindset, and the success rate is amazing. It was a blessing to learn from him. He was and is, to this day, a complete class act and wonderful man.

My training at this point in my young life became much more about strength and the three power lifts, as well as getting physically larger. It would be years before I would ever feel I had enough muscle to start the "sculpting" process. For now, I needed a foundation. Strength came easily to me. I started handling weights that many my size and age could not.

Before long, I was benching over 300lbs, squatting, and deadlifting over 400lbs as well. I started to do a bit of powerlifting, which consisted of those three lifts, bench, squat, and deadlifts. I still did a lot of bodybuilding exercises as well, but my main focus was the big three!

We live in a world where so much is not within our control. With weight training, you enter a world that is very black and white. For example, there is a barbell on the floor. It is loaded to weigh 405lbs. You have to deadlift it. Simple. You either can, or you can't. You can argue with that barbell all day long, and it won't matter. Succeed or fail. Black and white. If you failed, you could choose to continue to work, and eventually, you would succeed! For an individual that constantly struggled with everyday life, this endeavour became a lifesaver!

Olympik was my safe place. My church. My pastors and teachers were the owners and elite lifters. All under the watchful eyes of Ollie, his face forever straining with the huge weight he was holding. Ultimate focus. Olympik was my salvation.

CHAPTER 15

"You go, I go!"

One lesson I learned very well during my time at Olympik Gym was the importance of having a good training partner. Over the years, there have been times when I was forced to train alone because of the odd shifts I was working at the time. Having trained with a partner and by myself, I can honestly say that training with a partner helped me to push myself harder than when training alone.

My first real training partner was Paul Winter. We were the same age and often found ourselves training at the same time of day. Physically we were opposites. Although we were the same height and weighed about the same, our bodies developed quite differently. Paul was all back and shoulders. He had huge lats and naturally wide clavicles. When he wore a sweatshirt, he looked massive! Whereas I was limb dominant. My arms and legs were much more developed than my shoulders and back. If you could combine the two bodies, you would have had a very balanced physique! This was the main reason we started training together. Paul wanted to bring up his arms and legs, and I wanted to bring up my back and shoulders. We also got along really well and would constantly crack each other up during workouts as well as challenge each other to do more reps, more weight, and more sets!

Arnold was a big influence on both of us. We both did our best to master his Austrian accent, and we would often speak in "Arnold" through many of our workouts. I am quite sure that probably annoyed some of the other regulars. We were, of course, oblivious to this. It was one of the many ways we kept our training fun, and it also helped us to focus. In our minds, we were starring in our own version of "Pumping Iron." We had both seen the documentary so many times we could pretty much recite it word for word!

I had finally moved out of the "frat house" I had been sharing with the Klassen boys and Merv. My friend Rob's parents had developed the second story of their house into a bachelor suite, complete with a full kitchen and bathroom. When their tenant moved out, they offered it to me. It was a great place. I finally had my own space. Mrs. Kliewer often left fresh baking on the stairwell that led to my little pad, and they welcomed me to celebrate Christmas with them and treated me as part of the family. It felt like home.

More often than not, Paul would come by my little place before we would train. I would make us both a very calorie-dense protein shake. Since we were both trying to put on as much mass as possible, we were not afraid of calories. Not to mention that at our age, it seemed as though our bodies would soak up everything that we ate and turned it into muscle.

The shakes would often consist of mass gainer protein powder, whole milk, bananas, whole eggs, chocolate milk, and ice cream. They were delicious. How I wish that my metabolism was still like that! We would drink our cement shakes (as I called them) and discuss what we were going to train that day.

Paul did nothing halfway. He was an intense individual at that point in his life. I often felt like I had to watch out for him as he had a wild side, and I didn't want him to get arrested or get into trouble. In a million years, it never occurred to me that I would be the one that would end up on the wrong side of the law!

It was fun to have someone to compete with, and we were forever messing with each other.

One day, he called me before coming by to pick me up and asked, "Hey, you cool if Lisa comes with us today? She wants to train a bit. Don't worry, she won't be training with us," he laughed as he said it.

"Fine with me," I replied. I liked his girlfriend Lisa, so I thought nothing of it.

A few minutes later, he showed up, and I made us our cement shakes.

"Where's Lisa?" Paul smiled a smile that told me something was up.

"She's waiting in the truck." Again, that evil smile crossed his lips.

When we went downstairs to his truck, there was Lisa, all right, standing by the truck with an absolutely gorgeous blonde girl I had never seen before.

Paul started laughing and introduced us, "Todd, this is Lisa's friend Michelle."

I was caught totally off guard. This girl was stunning, and I was barely able to mumble out a hello. Paul's truck was small and had no backseat, just a bench seat in the front. It was like Paul was reading my mind, and before I could say anything about where we would all sit, he said, "Hey bro, Michelle is going to have to sit on your lap. You ok with that?"

He could barely contain his laughter as I struggled to say anything that made any sense. Normally I had no problem talking to girls, but for some reason, this girl intimidated me. She was a Goddess, and there was something about her that made me uncharacteristically nervous. Like a kid with a crush on his teacher is the best way to describe it. She just seemed so far out of my league.

Michelle looked at me and asked very sweetly, "Is that ok? That I sit on your lap?" All I could do was nod as I felt my face turn red. Paul and Lisa pretty much laughed the whole drive to the gym. I had this gorgeous girl sitting on my lap, and I'm wearing sweatpants, and the ride was not a smooth one.

One thought and one thought only was running through my mind as we drove, "Oh man, do NOT get excited now!!!" Once we got to the gym, the girls did their own thing, and Paul and I started to warm up.

"Thanks for the heads-up dickhead!" I said quietly enough so the girls wouldn't hear.

He could not stop laughing at me as he chuckled, "Man, I have NEVER seen you so flustered!!! She is ridiculously hot, though, hey?"

I had to agree on that point.

Then he continued, "Don't forget, there is the ride home yet! Hope you can control yourself!"

All I could reply was, "Control myself? Man, I can't even string together three words to say to her!"

We both laughed at that.

Needless to say, I had one of the best workouts of my life, as I am pretty sure Michelle had caused my testosterone levels to double just by being there!

We were very competitive in the gym. I had a slight edge in strength in most lifts; however, on back days, it was a different story. We were always trying to outdo one another; that was half the fun. When we trained, I would always make him perform the first set of every exercise so that I could watch him and gauge his energy levels.

Another advantage it gave me was that I always knew how many reps I had to complete to beat him. It would drive him mental. If he did ten reps, I did eleven. If he did twenty reps, I would do twenty-one. Even if I could do twenty-five, I would only do just ONE more to beat him. That would make him even madder.

He would always ask why I didn't do more, and my answer was always the same, "I only have to do one more than you! That's the way it goes, Paul. You go, I go! If you beat me, then it's I go, you go!"

That would cause him to push even harder, which in turn would push me as well. It was a great way to keep him motivated, and in turn, it helped my training. On the days we trained back, I was not so cocky. If my energy was down even a little bit, he would destroy me and, of course, taunt me the whole time! I expected nothing less. It was an all-out war when we trained, and that resulted in both of us growing in strength and size.

One of my favorite things to do when we trained was to get Paul laughing if he was getting close to beating me in a given exercise. On one occasion, when we were doing bench press, Paul was having a great day. He was keeping up with me set for set and rep for rep.

Normally I could beat him pretty easily on the bench, but on this particular day, he was really feeling great, and I was lagging. He started to taunt me a bit, "Today is the day you fall!"

This was, of course, completely unacceptable to me. Bench press was my best lift, after all. I could handle it when he beat me on a back exercise; I expected him to, as he was genetically gifted for back lifts. The bench was my baby.

Uncharacteristically, I kept quiet as we progressed, adding weight to each set until we were nearing the 300lb mark. He didn't know it, but I had a plan. Now that Paul was on his heaviest set, it was time to ensure that he would not do more reps than I could handle. He began his set, pressing the 300lb barbell easily. I counted out his reps aloud, "One, two, three, four, five, six."

Now it was time to sabotage him as I knew I was not getting much more than seven or eight reps at that weight on this day. As he started to press his seventh rep, I broke into my best Arnold accent, "Come on, Pauly, that weight is nothzing more zan a toothzpick with cheerios on ze ends!"

He broke out laughing, and the weight came crashing down on his barrel chest. Now I started laughing as well, and when you laugh, you have ZERO strength. Paul is now pinned under 300lbs, and he is laughing and trying to get the weight off his chest and into the rack, and I am pulling on the barbell and laughing so hard I am of little help. Some of the regulars started laughing as well, which made it worse. He is turning red from the pressure and laughter, and I can't do much to help him.

Finally, after many attempts, the two of us manage to rack the weight, and he starts chasing me around the gym, yelling in his best Arnold voice, "I'M GOING TO KEEEEL YOUUUU!!!" Once we catch our breath, it is my turn to press. Paul does his best to crack me up during my set, but I have my blinders on. He counts out the reps, "four, five, six, ah you prick. You're going to beat me, seven, eight, argh!"

With that, I rack the barbell and look at him, and in a quiet voice, I say, "I win." Then we both burst out laughing again.

When we finally stopped chuckling, he said, "It's not fair. You always know how many reps you have to beat!"

My reply was simple, "That's how it goes, Pauly. I won, so you go, I go."

CHAPTER 16

GI Blues

Since a very young age, I had held an admiration for the military. Perhaps it had something to do with the fact that I was fascinated with strength and power. The uniforms, the honour, the tradition. All of it really spoke to me. One of my favorite movies was "The Dirty Dozen," which I had watched every time it was shown on late-night TV. It was about a group of incarcerated soldiers during WW2. They were given a chance at freedom if they "volunteered" for a suicide mission deep behind German enemy lines. I could picture myself as one of these soldiers. The thought of doing something brave and admirable really spoke to me.

Since I really wasn't doing anything meaningful in terms of education or career, the thought of entering the military, specifically the Army, was starting to enter my thoughts on a frequent basis. There was nothing to lose. "How tough could it be?" was my train of thought. I started talking to my friend Trevor about the idea. His father had been in the Army. He decided to come down with me to the recruiting office to check it out. Once there, we got some basic information, and the recruiting NCO suggested that we watch a video on the Canadian Armed Forces. The video talked about the grand history of our military, different careers available, and then showed a glimpse of basic training. The basic training stood out the most. It looked scary, intense. Challenging. It frightened me, which of course, meant I had to join. After we left, both a little shell-shocked from watching the rigors of Army training, I asked Trevor, "what do you think? Want to do it?" He looked at me like I had lost my marbles. "No chance!" was his reply. Trevor was much more of a thinker, kind-hearted to a fault. There was nothing he saw in that video that appealed to him. All I could see was the challenge as well as a way out of being a nobody. I enlisted.

Joining the Army is not as easy as I had imagined. There was quite the process involved: a basic physical (turn your head and cough, please), eyesight requirements, hearing tests, an aptitude test, as well as an in-depth interview. This was all a surprise to me. Television and movies had led me to believe that if you could walk and chew gum, they wanted you! Thousands of dollars went into the training of each soldier. The Canadian Armed Forces took recruiting very seriously. They wanted the best they could find.

As a recruit, you are given three choices as to what trade you wanted to take. Being very gung-ho, all of my choices were combat arms. Soldiering. My first choice was Armoured, as in tanks. Arnold Schwarzenegger had been a tank driver in the Austrian Army, and I wanted to follow in his footsteps. My second choice was Infantry, a real grunt, a soldier. The third choice was an Artilleryman, canons. After going through all the interviews and jumping through many hoops, I was informed that because I did not have my grade 12 diploma, they had nothing to offer me at that time. However, should I complete Grade 12, there could possibly be a spot for me in the Canadian Armed Forces. I assured the recruiting NCO that I would complete my Grade 12, and with a handshake, I was on my way. I registered for night classes immediately and was determined to finally get my diploma from high school. Even though there was no ceremony, it had always bothered me that I had not graduated. So, when I received my GED certificate, it felt like a weight had been lifted off of my shoulders.

Several months went by, and no word from the Recruiting Center. I had almost forgotten about the Army altogether and was trying to figure out what to do next with my life. Then one day, out of the blue, the Army called. The recruiting NCO asked me over the phone if I had completed my grade 12. Once we got that out of the way, he went on to explain that there was an opening for my third career option, Artilleryman. He then asked if I would accept that position or wait for my first or second choice? I was thrilled. Of course, I would accept. It sounded like the beginning of a grand adventure. I would be a SOLDIER! In my mind, I would make my mother proud of me. I was doing something with honour and purpose. Serving my country. I could not wait. My training was to start in a few weeks at CFB Cornwallis in Nova Scotia. If it had been up to me, I would have started the next day.

In the few weeks, before I was to be shipped off to basic training, I spent my time saying goodbye to all the friends that mattered to me. My girlfriend at the time, Vittoria, was deeply saddened by the thought of me leaving. I tried to break up with her as I did not see how we could continue being a couple with me being so far away. She was my first serious girlfriend, and we were convinced we were in love. She simply refused to break up, so we decided we would remain a couple and would stay in touch and see each other whenever I had leave. She knew which buttons to push to make me listen to my heart and not logic.

Finally, the day came. Fittingly, Trevor offered to drive me to the airport. I had said goodbye to Rob Kliewer and all the guys I had grown up with, and it was time to go. All I packed was my gym bag. In it were my gym clothes and basic toiletries. I was hopeful that the Army would allow me to continue to lift weights.

Saying goodbye to Trevor was much harder than I had imagined. We had been through a lot. He had been a very loyal friend, sticking by me in my worst times and listening to me ramble on into the wee hours of the night on many occasions. We laughed together, sang old songs together, and tried to chase girls together.

In many ways, Trevor and Rob had been more like family to me than anyone else. He gave me a lift to the airport in his old beat-up car, and we tried to talk as we always did. This time it felt different. Sad. When it was time for me to go, he gave me a big hug as we both teared up. In retrospect, I think we both realized that not only were we saying goodbye to each other, but also, we were saying goodbye to our childhoods.

Thus, my little Army adventure began. To this point, I had only been out of Manitoba twice in my life and had never been on an airplane. The speed the plane attained on the runway blew my mind as I peered out the window in amazement like an excited little kid. Before take-off, I had visions of perhaps one day being a paratrooper and jumping out of airplanes into dangerous territories. That all changed as the plane gained altitude. As I looked out of the window, I realized that jumping out of a perfectly good airplane sounded a lot better in my head. As I watched the ground get farther and farther away as we climbed, the dream of being a paratrooper quickly disappeared.

As luck would have it, I was seated next to a very pleasant young French woman from St. Boniface who was also on her way to basic training. Her name was Nicole. Neither one of us really had any idea what was awaiting us in Cornwallis. It was very comforting to have her as a travelling companion as we were both more than a little nervous. We passed the time with silly jokes and conversations about what we thought basic training would be like.

Finally, we arrived in Halifax. Once I departed the plane, an odd thought struck me: I had absolutely no idea where I was going or what the next step was! All I knew was that I was to board this flight from Winnipeg to Halifax. I asked Nicole if she had any clue as to what we were supposed to do now. Same as me, her only instructions were to be on that plane. So here I was, at an airport, far from home and quite clueless!

We wandered around the airport looking for anyone that looked like they were connected with the military. After a short time, we began to notice other young men and women wandering around with the same lost expressions. After talking to a few of them, it was quite clear we were all in the same boat.

I decided to go to the information desk to see if I could find out anything.

"Excuse me, Miss," I asked, " I am from Winnipeg, and I am here to begin my basic training with the Canadian Armed Forces. Do you have information regarding recruits being picked up?"

A sly smile crossed her lips as she answered, "Don't worry, this happens every week. They will come and get you. It might take a while. Just relax."

She was chuckling as she said it. So, we proceeded to hurry up and wait. Some of the recruits decided to go to the airport bar and have a few drinks. This turned out to be a bad idea. I passed the time by chatting with other recruits. Hours passed, still nothing. I was getting tired, hungry, and agitated. By this time, some of the recruits were drunk.

Then it happened. Several buses came rolling up. Once stopped, the doors opened, and out came several very intimidating-looking NCOs (Non-Commissioned Officers). They were all business and quickly began rounding all the recruits up like cattle and lining us up into formation. They ordered us to stand at attention. Precise and quiet, all of this happened with very little noise. Instead of shouting instructions, they whispered commands into our ears which was much more frightening.

Once they had all the stragglers from the bar lined up, they marched us onto the buses. It was now 11:00 pm. We were all tired, and most of us were pretty scared. Once we were all loaded on the buses, the quiet whispers turned into yelling. The drunk guys got the worst of it. I sat in the back, trying to hide. Seated next to me was a thinly built blond guy by the name of Peters. I do not remember his first name as we were not allowed to use first names when addressing each other. We told each other that we would get through this, and we would stick together. Safe to say, we were both scared and realized that the training video we had watched had left out a lot of details about basic training.

The bus lumbered on through the night, and I noticed that we were driving up and down many hills. It seemed as though we were going downhill much more than we were going up. I leaned over and quietly whispered to Peters, "Hey, you notice that we seem to be going mostly downhill?" "Yeah," he answered. "That's because we are heading to Hell!" We both laughed at that and were promptly scolded by the NCO.

Once we had arrived at CFB Cornwallis, we were herded into our barracks. Two-story, "H" shaped buildings. We were commanded to stand in front of our bunks and then ordered to empty our bags so they could inspect our personal belongings for drugs and illegal items.

Out of the corner of my eye, I could see that the recruit next to me was obviously into weight training as he was quite muscular. I also noticed that he sported a short ponytail. One by one, the NCOs inspected our belongings and found excuses to yell at various recruits for the smallest of reasons.

When they got to the fellow next to me, I heard the NCO exclaim, "What do we have here? A ponytail? He then began to go through the recruit's personal belongings and began laughing loudly, and called over two other NCOs. "Boys, take a look at this!!!" he chortled. In his belongings were a large amount of hair care products. Gel, shampoo, hair spray, mousse. "Looks like recruit thinks he's at beauty school!"

With that remark, the recruit rolled his eyes. Big mistake! All hell broke loose as the three NCOs began yelling at him at once—one in each ear and one in his face. They commanded him to hit the ground and start doing push-ups. I stopped counting after 50. They made him do push-ups until he could no longer move an inch. His name was Bensimmon. He had a definite knack for getting into trouble, as I was to later find out. After the inspections were over, we were allowed to finally go to bed. I was completely exhausted.

Day one started with a bang quite literally. With no warning, the NCOs stormed into the barracks hitting garbage can lids with batons and yelling for us to get up! I was so startled I fell off the top bunk and was immediately ordered to perform 25 push-ups for being so stupid. The day was spent getting us organized with all of our kits. We each received a footlocker, uniforms, labels, boots, berets, and everything a soldier would need.

We were then marched off to receive our official Army haircuts. I wasn't particularly stressed about the haircut as I was already sporting a brush-cut. Then the first recruit came out of the base barbershop, we all gasped. He was pretty much bald. All that was left on his head was some stubble on top. When it was my turn, I was surprised to find out we had to pay for these great haircuts, $3.50! The barber used a straight razor and was deaf. I thought to myself, if he cuts me, he won't even hear me yell! When he was finished, the image I saw in the mirror shocked me. My brush-cut was long compared to this scalping!

The next few weeks were spent learning the fundamentals of being a soldier. We learned how to take care of our kit. Polishing boots, ironing uniforms, sewing labels by hand onto every single piece of kit we were issued. These tasks were to be performed in the evening after supper was served. During the day, it was mostly marching, PT (physical training) as well as some classroom lessons. Everything was strictly regimented. What I did not realize at the time is that we were being trained to respond to orders without questioning anything. They systematically broke us down only to rebuild us as soldiers.

Up until this point in my life, I had thought I had the ability to push myself very hard in terms of physical tasks or training. This was a whole new level. I wasn't used to so many things being out of my control. Everything we did in basic had to be perfect. All done on minimal sleep. The physical training was quite intense.

I remember quite vividly the day that we did our run test. There were certain physical standards that each recruit had to meet. One of the tests was a mile and a half run. You had to be able to run it in under 12 minutes. The day of the run, we were all getting changed into our gym clothes when I noticed a recruit from another unit, his name was Tanner, and I knew him from Winnipeg. He saw me as well and made his way over. It was great seeing someone from home. We only had a few minutes to chat as I changed. He was two weeks ahead of me on the course.

"Have you done the run test yet?" he asked.

"No, we are doing it today."

His eyes widened with his reply, "Whatever you do, run slow! Seriously man, go slow!!!"

With that, he had to leave as his platoon NCO had shown up and was yelling at them all to get a move on and report to the parade square right quick. I did not have a chance to ask him why he told me to run slow. I wasn't worried, a mile and a half run was not a big deal for me at the time, and like every physical challenge, I decided to do my best and ignore Tanner's advice. My time was fast, well under ten minutes. Not the fastest, but certainly in the top group.

"That was easy," I thought to myself.

A valuable lesson was about to be learned the next time we had PT (physical training). As we lined up in our ranks, Master Corporal Pedrosa started calling our names and putting us into three different groups. My group consisted of all of the guys that had finished with the fastest times. A very fit NCO was put in charge of my group, and off we went for our run.

Again, I was not worried as the first run had been easy. The Master Corporal led us to the base of a steep hill. A bad feeling started to form in my gut as we began running uphill. This was definitely not something I was used to. Manitoba is largely flat as a pancake. I had zero experience running hills. There were, of course, the stairs I used to run when training for both basketball and boxing, but I hadn't trained like that since I started lifting weights and was now at least twenty pounds heavier than those days.

It was a steep incline. Up and down, he ran us, over and over. He was in tremendous physical condition as he ran with us the whole way. Unlike the recruits (myself included), he never got out of breath. My legs were starting to burn, and my lungs were working very hard to get enough air to continue. All the while, the NCO not only ran, he also shouted a continuous stream of insults as we all started falling behind. Some of the guys started falling down in exhaustion, a few puked.

The NCO (he was called a Physical Training Instructor) would run back to the fallen, yell at them to get up, and then would still have enough energy to catch up to the lead group. Up until that point, I had thought I was in good shape. This instructor was clearly not human, was the thought running through my head. He made me feel pitiful by comparison. My only victory that day was that I completed the run. Barely. Only a few of us managed this task. Every time we would run, this instructor devised a different way to torture us.

Later, I found out that if you qualified to be in the fast group, they ran you to death every time to make us even faster. The guys that had trouble with the run test were brought along slowly to get their endurance up to par. The next time I saw Tanner, he asked me how the run went and if I had run slow as he advised.

"I ran fast," I answered sheepishly.

He laughed extremely hard at that and, in between chuckles, said, "You are a dumbass! Did you make it into the fast group?"

I nodded. He laughed even harder.

As the weeks went by, it became clear that some of the recruits were not cut out for Military life. We were tested to our limits both physically and mentally. One day during lunch, we all stared in amazement as one recruit had decided that he had quite enough of the Army and basic training, and in his full combat uniform, he started walking into the Bay as we sat eating our lunch. The mess hall overlooked this body of water, so there was no missing it. If this was a suicide attempt, it was certainly not a pleasant one as that water would have been close to the freezing point. I felt bad for the two MPs that were sent in to drag him out. He was sent home that week with a dishonourable discharge.

The Army had some very interesting ideas in regard to motivating us. One incident I will never forget was the day they took us to the pool for our swim test. We were instructed to report to the pool in our full combat gear, except for our boots. Under our uniforms, we wore our swim trunks, which were Speedo's.

The NCOs lined up all the recruits beside the pool and began explaining the task that was to be performed. Standing in front of me were two Inuit brothers from another unit in our platoon. They were whispering to each other and look decidedly nervous. Just as I was about to ask what was wrong, one of the brothers turned to me and quietly muttered, "Hey, Payette, we got a big problem."

"What's up?" I replied.

"We can't swim!"

I remember thinking to myself, "Oh crap."

I spent the next several minutes trying to teach the two brothers how to swim, or should I say, trying to EXPLAIN to them how to swim. They had no pools in their village, and of course, the water there was way too cold to swim in.

Finally, it was time for the first brother to begin his swim test. Each of us was to jump off of a three-meter diving board, then tread water for several minutes, then swim to the end of the pool and back and again tread water for another few minutes. Brother number one was now standing at the end of the diving board awaiting his command to jump.

"RECRUIT JUMP!" the NCO shouted.

Brother number one hit the water and sank like a stone. Through much effort, he managed to struggle to the surface. It was obvious he was in trouble and panicking and had forgotten any instructions on swimming I had tried to convey. We all watched in horror as he struggled to stay afloat.

The only help he received from the NCO was one word that the NCO shouted over and over, "SWIM!"

This was the Army's version of how to motivate an individual. They waited until it was obvious he was going to drown, and then they fished him out. Once out of the pool, the NCO proceeded to berate brother number one on his incompetence as he sputtered and coughed up pool water.

It was now brother number two's turn. He was now shaking in fear. We all felt horrible for him. Now at the end of the diving board, the NCO gave the command to jump. The brother did not move. The NCO repeated himself, "RECRUIT JUMP!!" Still, he remained motionless. The NCO's face was turning red as he yelled, " RECRUIT! YOU BETTER JUMP INTO THE FUCKING WATER RIGHT NOW, OR I WILL COME UP THERE AND PERSONALLY KICK YOUR ASS INTO THE POOL!!!" Again, another fine example of the Army's motivational methodology.

With that, brother number two jumped. It played out exactly the same as it had for his brother. They were both ordered to report to remedial swim. Now it was my turn. Although I was a bit shaken up by what I had witnessed, the test did not worry me as I was a decent enough swimmer. HOWEVER, while trying to instruct the two brothers on the finer points of swimming, I had missed out on a very crucial bit of information given out during the instructions. That key bit of info was simple, button your pants up as tight as you could.

"RECRUIT JUMP!"

I hit the water and bobbed to the surface, and began to tread water. The first thing I noticed was that treading water in full combats was not easy. The material of the uniform was very heavy when wet. The second thing I noticed was that my pants kept falling down. After what seemed like an eternity, I received the command to swim to the end of the pool. This was easier said than done, as my pants were down around my knees. I could barely move. My solution was to take my pants off. I balled them up as best as I could and completed the swim test with my pants in one hand. Every second stroke I took was very ridiculous looking as the balled-up pants would hit the water like a bowling ball. SPLOOOSH, stroke, SPLOOSH, stroke.

He called over two other NCOs to watch. Once I completed the test, they ordered me out of the pool, and I put my pants back on. In between fits of laughter, the NCO finally asked me, "What in the name of baby Jesus was that?"

I quietly explained my pants kept falling off. I was ordered to report to remedial swim along with the two brothers.

Remedial swim was pretty much what you would expect. Simply put, they were teaching recruits how to swim. How to hold your breath, tread water, and so on. By the third class, we were instructed to try to swim to the end of the pool. Unlike the others, I knew how to swim and was only there because I was an idiot. When it was my turn, I dove into the pool and calmly swam to the other side, turned around, and swam back. Once out of the pool, the NCO asked me why I was in remedial swim as it was evident that I was a decent swimmer. As I told him my swim test story, he began to laugh harder and harder. After I finished regaling him with my sad tale, he instructed me that I was no longer required to attend remedial swim.

As the weeks passed, I was slowly transformed into a soldier. Gas warfare training, obstacle courses, weapons training, hand-to-hand combat, as well as what seemed like endless marching and drill were part of our daily routine. The weeks passed by, and thankfully, basic training came to a close.

After basic, we were sent to CFB Shilo to begin Battle School. There I was to receive the training I needed to be an actual Artilleryman. What I did not realize was that my military stint was to be cut short. During a routine physical, it was discovered that both of my knees were pretty much shot. I knew this but kept it to myself. By the time I was done with high school sports, I felt pain in both knees whenever I ran or jumped. Through weightlifting, I had made the muscles strong enough that I could still perform at a high level. As far as I was concerned. I had no problems.

The Military Doctor had other ideas. Upon hearing the snap, crackle and popping sounds my knees made, my days as a soldier came to a screeching halt. The Canadian Armed Forces did give me the option of re-mustering into another trade, such as a clerk. To me at the time, this was not an option. I had joined to become a soldier, not a desk jockey. I was offered a medical discharge. They were sending me home.

All in all, the military was a great experience for me. Never in my life had I been pushed so hard. To this day, I am grateful for the experience. At the time, though, it was a huge disappointment. Again, I was in limbo. I had no idea what I was going to do. Upon arriving back in Winnipeg, I realized I had nowhere to go.

For some reason, I decided to go home to my Mom's. Once there, I explained what had happened with the military and my medical discharge. I swallowed my pride and asked if I could stay at home until I found a job and a place. She allowed me to stay only that night and was instructed I had to leave in the morning—that hurt. In hindsight, she did the right thing. I was not a child. I was a young man. It was time to grow up and get a move on with life.

The next morning, I packed up my meager gym bag and, for the second time, left home. I thought to myself, "Ok, soldier, here we go again. Let's see what you are made of!"

CHAPTER 17

Love and Marriage

Once my short-lived military career was over, it was time to go about the business of getting on with life. I still had my dreams, which now, more than ever, were about the bodybuilding world. In the meantime, I needed an income and a place to stay. The place to stay could not have worked out better. My friend Rob's parents, the Kliewers, had converted the second story of their home into a little apartment complete with its own kitchen and bathroom. It was $200.00 a month. Rob was still living with his folks in the basement, which was great as we often hung out. Not to mention Mrs. Kliewer often left fresh baking for me on the steps leading to my little pad.

I had resumed training at Olympik Gym and worked at various jobs to get by. I was given my job back at Olympik, which paid next to nothing. However, it allowed me to work at a place that I adored. It was not hard to make extra money doing security work.

My girlfriend Vittoria and I picked up things where we had left off. What I didn't know was that I was going to slowly walk away from my dreams and begin living my life like it was predetermined and beyond mundane.

My dream was to move to Southern California, the Mecca of Bodybuilding. In my head, it seemed simple enough. Move there, train, and learn all the secrets from the greatest bodybuilders on earth while working in a gym. Until, of course, I became Mr. Universe, that is!

As time went by, I let life get in the way. Vittoria wanted NO part of me moving away or my bodybuilding dreams. She was ok with me training, especially at Olympik, as there were almost no women there. Yet, she would constantly ask me who was in the gym after my workouts and would always grill me about the women that trained there, even though they were mostly wives and girlfriends of other members.

It's not that I blame Vitt for squashing my dreams. I hate when people blame their spouses or partners for not achieving their goals. Being accountable is hard, after all. The reason I did not pursue my goals at that time was simple; I was not strong enough to do so. Even though I had become very confident in certain areas of my life, in other aspects, I had very little belief in myself. Vittoria was loyal. That meant a lot to me. I chose to push my dreams to the side and began setting about the task of obtaining a completely average life. It became increasingly important to me that I made Vittoria and her family happy and proud of me.

Vittoria's family was Italian. Her mother had passed away from cancer when she was 13. This affected her deeply. She had an older brother Tony, and they lived with her "Pa," Joe. Her grandmother, who everyone referred to as "Nana," lived directly across the street from them and often spent the night. Her husband, or "Nono," had passed away years earlier.

Joe was an ex-professional wrestler and was about five foot eight. What he lacked in height, he made up for in width and tenacity. Joe was a real man. He did not take shit from anyone. I liked him immediately. He still worked the wrestling circuit as a referee, and his full-time job was as a sales rep for a dairy. Over time we became close. I loved talking boxing with him, and I always felt he respected that I trained and had boxed. He could eat ridiculous amounts of pasta yet always remained in pretty decent shape.

During supper, he would often eat with no shirt on and slap his chest as wrestlers do. The first meal I shared with them almost killed me. I could eat, don't get me wrong. However, the first bowl of pasta they put on the table was so large I assumed it was for everyone.

Vittoria must have realized what I was thinking as she leaned over and whispered, "That bowl is for Pa."

The amount of pasta they gave me was insane. I got the feeling it was a test. Sort of like, "This is how a man eats, so you better finish it!" I made sure I ate it all and felt ten pounds heavier by the time I was done.

If you happened to go across the street to Nana's, one would have to be prepared to eat. Hungry or not, Nana would offer you food in her broken English.

"You wanna mangiare?"

If you politely refused, she would say, "Please, mangiare just a poco?" Which means eat just a little. If you refused, she would kind of cry. She was forever offering a Sprite to drink with it. She wanted to make sure no one ever left hungry. In fact, the first time I ever dieted down to get ripped, she hated it. I would not eat pasta, and she thought I was dying.

Joe trained a bit in his house with equipment and benches he made by himself out of wood. Some days I would train there as well and was always amazed at how sturdy those wooden benches were. He later made me a bed frame that I wish I still had as it was solid as granite!

Vittoria's brother Tony also used the weights on occasion. He was like a super-sized version of his father: five-foot-ten and easily 260lbs with the widest set of shoulders I had seen on a person to that point in my life. He was as intelligent as he was big. He got straight A's in high school and University. He was not a person to be taken lightly. In high school, he once beat up a substitute teacher that made a derogatory remark about his mother. The teacher made reference to Tony's manners being subpar and that his mother obviously didn't teach him anything.

The teacher did not realize at the time that Tony's mother was dying of cancer. Tony simply went right at him and kicked his ass. I believe that was the last time he ever taught at that school. I did not fear Tony. I liked him. He could be funny as hell, and because he had zero fear, he had some hilarious stories to tell. That being said, I had no wish to ever mess with him.

Only once did we get into an argument that ended in me telling Tony to go fuck himself. This was at the dinner table, we both leapt up out of our chairs, and Joe got in between us. Tony was used to people backing down. That was not something I was prepared to do. I did, of course, realize that if we came to blows, we were both going to suffer big damage. With Joe holding us apart, I told Vitt to get her coat, and we left.

The next day, one of the tires on my little Pontiac Acadian was slashed. When I told Vitt, she said only one thing, "Tony!" She told me the next time I saw him to pay attention to how he acted towards me. She said, "If he is super nice to you, he for sure slashed your tire. It's his way of covering it up."

Sure enough, the next time I saw him, he was sweet as can be. She knew her brother. Tony and I never had a disagreement after that day.

Time continued to march on. I fell into a routine. I morphed into being part of Vittoria's family and their way of doing things. I found a job at a steel shop and, for the first time in my life, was making a decent wage. At least it seemed to be at the time. The $12.93/hour was double the wage I had ever made before. The company even paid for me to take welding classes at night so I would have a trade, and this also gave me some job protection when work got slow. They tried not to lay off their skilled workers as there was always that chance that they would find jobs elsewhere, which meant hiring new staff and training them.

Once I had my welding tickets, my wage increased to over $17.00/hour. I felt rich. My dreams slipped further away. I was doing what I was "supposed" to do. This was what a man did. I wanted the people in my life to be proud of me even though deep inside, a little piece of me was dying.

I was welding galvanized steel. The fumes were very toxic. We wore respirators, and that helped to a degree. The shop was not ventilated very well, and I found myself getting sick on a regular basis. I had discovered I had mild asthma, and the longer I welded, the worse it got. Each day I would wake up and spend 20 minutes in the bathroom expelling crud from my lungs. It was awful. Bodybuilding and California moved into the land of my dreams as I forged ahead trying to do the "right things."

Years had passed. I was in my twenties but was living like a middle-aged man: work, gym, home, and repeat. Empty best describes how I felt. For the life of me, I could not figure out why I was not happy. At the time, doing the right thing also meant getting married. After all, Vittoria had been loyal to me for five years now. Yes, she could be jealous and controlling. We often fought. I knew no different. I wanted her to be happy, her Pa and Nana to be happy. Also, I thought it would make my mother proud. I drove Vitt to the park where I had first asked her to be my girlfriend and proposed, giving her my mother's engagement ring.

A wedding is a wonderful way to distract yourself from the fact that you are, in fact, miserable. We had the wedding social to arrange, the dress, tuxedo, the actual wedding. It's the biggest party ever, and it was all for us! It made me feel like a man. I would have a wife. I was a welder. A big guy. This was success, was it not? The wedding was large in my mind, with about 150 guests. We were married in a Catholic Church, of course. Small for an Italian wedding, though.

The reception was at the Fort Garry Hotel, a gorgeous historic hotel in Winnipeg. The food was amazing with every Italian Pastry you could imagine. The highlight of the night for me was giving a short speech. I spoke about Vittoria's family and meeting them for the first time. About Joe's enormous pasta bowl and chest smacking like an Italian gorilla. People laughed as they had all witnessed Joe in all his glory at one time or another. That speech was given out of love. I loved these people. Yet, I was unhappy. Something was missing.

There were two things that really made me wonder if I was doing the right thing. During the ceremony, as Vittoria was walking down the aisle, I felt zero emotion. By nature, I am romantic and emotional. It was odd to me that my bride was standing beside me, and I felt nothing. She also had no tears of joy, no emotion. This wasn't what I expected. The second thing that struck me as odd was that the only time Vittoria showed any emotion was after her dance with her father. She cried as they finished. I remember thinking, "Zero emotion towards me, but crying at the thought of leaving her Dad." Deep down, it didn't feel right.

We lived in a few little apartments before buying a small bi-level house in a newer neighborhood. As best as I could, I continued to try and do the "right things." We got a little Chocolate Lab Puppy and named her Thea. Joe and I landscaped the yard. It was a cute little house. It was as though I was trying to live the Norman Rockwell ideal. We took a couple of trips to Vegas, three in fact. It was a distraction.

As time passed, a slow realization began to grip me. This was not my life. Average would not work for me on any level. It wasn't that I felt better than anyone or above anyone. That wasn't it at all. Deep down, I knew that an "ordinary life" would not cut it for me, and I would end up like my father, dead in the garage with the car running.

One day after work, as I sat in my new car, the song "Purple Rain" by Prince came on the radio. It was a huge hit when I was in high school. Hearing the haunting melody, I felt transported back to those days. I had dreams of becoming a Champion, dreams of California. It hit me like a rock. I sobbed. It was time to change it all, or I would die. I had to break the heart of a woman that never did anything wrong to me. I had to disappoint all the people that had been there for me. I was living someone else's life and was having thoughts of ending my own existence. I knew deep down that I had to start over. To that point, it was one of the toughest decisions of my life. It was on me. I had failed.

Once again, I would start over.

CHAPTER 18

Lost in Limbo

Alone. Single. This was definitely uncharted territory for me. Often, I had fantasized about it, dreamt of it. Now here I was, by myself. Vittoria and I had been together for almost 13 years. Since we were both in our teens, it felt as though I had not even had a period in my life that was my twenties. My existence had been that of a much older man. It wasn't that I felt I had missed out on partying or women; it was just that I had always had someone to answer to. Now it was just me, and it felt very foreign.

Career-wise, I made a change. The smoke was taking its toll on my lungs, along with the monotony of production welding. When I looked at the older fellows in my shop, they all shared a look of hopelessness. They looked tired and worn out. No one spoke of dreams or goals. They were like zombies waiting to die. This was not the life I wanted. There had to be more, and I certainly did not want to be sitting on an overturned paint pail, eating bologna sandwiches waiting for the lunch buzzer to sound so I could go back to work when I was 58 years old.

Other than working out, I really didn't have any marketable skills, so to speak, except one. I could talk. Communication had long been my strong suit, and I found that for some reason, I could converse with almost anyone and get them to open up. My friends suggested I look into being a salesperson. What to sell was the question. Real estate, furniture, electronics, none of these products interested me, so I decided to try Auto Sales. Cars are something that people are often passionate about. I still remembered buying my first new car and being extremely pumped at the time. Emotions, that was something that spoke to me. There was something I had to make peace with first. The stereotype of the car salesman really bothered me. However, there was a new car model that gave me hope. SATURN was a newer line from General Motors that had an interesting marketing strategy, no haggling. The price was the price. The sales process then became about looking after the customer. No pressure.

As it turns out, it is not very difficult to get a job selling cars. I literally went to the nearest Saturn dealer and asked to speak with the Sales Manager. After speaking with him, he decided to give me a shot. This dealership was part of a large dealer group, and they had all new prospective Salespeople go through a training course. Once you completed that, you were on the floor selling cars. So, there I was, waiting around a car dealership waiting for customers to come in. We were like sharks, really. Some guys hung out on the lot. Others hid at their desks. Or congregate in what was known in the car business as the "dope ring." Managers hated dope rings. It is when a group of salespeople stand around and basically just talk about nothing or bitch about how awful the car biz really is or complain about customers.

The list of things to complain about can be long. After all, it's a really ridiculous industry. Even without the haggling on the price of new vehicles, we were, of course, under the gun to sell. The no haggling did not really apply to the used cars on our lot, or "pre-owned" as dealerships like to call them. So, there was that whole song and dance with customers to contend with. The whole back and forth between customers and Sales Managers is really a silly outdated way of doing business.

Like any business, you have good bosses and not-so-good bosses. As a rule, most of the managers I worked under were pretty good, with a few exceptions. I often found myself selling more to my bosses than the customers.

Everyone has to find their own style when it comes to sales. I decided to completely ignore every sales technique they tried to teach me in their sales course. My strategy was simple, treat people how you would like to be treated. Be nice. That was it. It did not mean I could not ask customers for the sale or ask the tough questions. By the time we got to that point, I had earned the right to do so by simply communicating with them and getting to know them. Rapport was everything I was to find out. Of course, there were some individuals that I simply could not win over and some I did not want to. As it turns out, there are some people that are not worth having as customers. They will never be happy, even if they get a great car at a great price. Something would always bother them, and you would be the person they come to. It was easy enough to steer these folks in the direction of the door.

It turns out that simply being nice and treating people well goes a long way. In my very first month, I made more money selling cars than I had ever made welding. Perhaps I was onto something! Money has a way of covering up problems temporarily. So, for a while, I felt like I was succeeding. Working out was still a part of my life, but my dreams of being a champion bodybuilder were fading into my subconscious as I tried my best to be a superstar salesperson. I had started dating again and became involved in a few relationships. I preferred relationships rather than casual dating. Closeness was important to me. Being loved was very much something I longed for. There was, however, a realization that if a relationship ended, life would continue on. This was a lesson that was taught to me by a woman named Lisa.

A blind date? I had never been on a blind date. It was a customer of mine that had asked me if I was single. I had moved to a Honda dealership in our dealer group as SATURN had started to tank and eventually went out of business. Throughout our dealings, she had been very friendly with me and told me she had a girlfriend that I should meet if I was up for it. She arranged for me to call her, and our first communication was by phone. She was very charming and had a sense of humour, and was clearly very intelligent.

We decided to meet for coffee. I arrived first. We had decided to meet at a trendy outdoor café on Corydon, which was kind of a little Italy area of town. When she approached and said my name, I recognized her immediately. Lisa was a local celebrity that was an entertainment reporter for one of our news stations. She was tall and blond with a Hollywood smile and a charisma I had never encountered before in any woman I had dated. We shook hands, and she joined me. We hit it off immediately.

After finishing our drinks, I suggested we go to dinner, and off we went to a little Italian restaurant up the street. We found it easy to converse with each other, and we shared an offbeat sense of humour. She told me later that it was my ability to poke fun at myself that really attracted her to me. She had watched me arrive at the coffee place from her car to scope me out.

When she had seen that I was muscular, she almost pulled the plug right then and there. Asking her why, she replied, "Because most built guys are assholes."

Over dinner, I had broken into my impression of Arnold Schwarzenegger, totally mocking myself. It was at that moment that she really decided she liked me. As for myself, it was odd at first sitting across from a woman that I had watched on TV for years. She rolled with the successful people. In politics, entertainment, business, it seemed that she knew everyone. Wherever we went, we got the best table or best seats. People treated her amazingly well. What I came to realize was that she was just Lisa. A very charming, attractive, and intelligent woman that had her share of flaws, just like the rest of us. She was great to me. I was to learn a lot from her.

In some ways, my life was becoming almost surreal. I was making more money than I had ever seen in my life, and my girlfriend was a well-known entertainment reporter as well as a producer and was the host of our local jazz radio station's morning show.

Looking in the mirror, I still saw this rough kid from Elmwood. Dreams of becoming a Mr. Universe had vanished. Instead, I attended parties at rich people's houses. Invite only events, jazz concerts. We ate in the best places, and she never made me feel like I was anything but her partner or equal, except once. She would often talk to me about achieving more. In her opinion, I was selling myself short selling cars. She said I had a natural presence and that when we went to events, people would notice me, that I stood out. Coming from her, it was a huge compliment. After all, she had been to the Oscars, and she had interviewed Tom Cruise, Keanu Reeves, everyone really. It never occurred to me that being a car salesman might be a source of embarrassment to her. Although, to be perfectly honest, I never felt terribly comfortable telling people I was a "car salesman." The stigma was real.

We were dining at a lovely restaurant one evening when a heavyset gentleman approached our table exclaiming, "Lisa, how are you?" His arms were extended, and she stood up and hugged him, and they began to chat. Several minutes went by, and I began to feel self-conscious. She was clearly impressed by this man, and I could tell that he was one of the "important" people in her eyes. Finally, he looked over at me as one would examine a piece of steak in a butcher shop. It was then that Lisa realized she had not introduced me.

Her next statement made it quite clear to me that she did not want to introduce me. She simply stated, "Oh, I'm sorry, this is my FRIEND Todd."

"FRIEND?!? Since when am I a friend?" was the thought that raced through my mind. We had been dating exclusively for several months at this point. I was embarrassed. I stood up and grabbed the portly fellow's outstretched hand and shook it hard enough to make him wince. They exchanged a few more words as I sat down and resumed eating. They hugged, and he departed. The silence was deafening.

I said nothing.

She said nothing.

I looked at her. She knew she had messed up. Finally, I said one word very quietly, "friend."

She began to apologize profusely. "I don't know why I said that Todd, I am so sorry. Of course, you are more than a friend. You are my boyfriend, my partner."

I replied, "I know why you said it. You are embarrassed of me. I am not important; I am not in that circle of people. You are embarrassed to be with me."

She assured me that was not the case. Sadly, I think that moment was not one I could get past. It reinforced something I feared already. I was still just this nobody from Elmwood. It was these insecurities that would lead to Lisa and I eventually breaking up. We stayed together for a year and still had many amazing times. To this day, we are friends.

During this period, I learned something very important from Lisa. She put the idea back into my head that I was meant for something more, that I was not normal. Lisa thought maybe I would be good at marketing or some career other than car sales.

As time passed, I realized that money, fancy parties, even a trip to Asia, a nice car, none of that guaranteed happiness. These were all great things that most people aspired to have.

Inside I was empty. I was living a lie. I was barely working out anymore. I had no dreams of my own. In some ways, I felt like Lisa's escort to events. I was tired of fancy eateries. I wanted to lift weights and be an animal. Make love at the drop of a hat. Live life and laugh hard and love hard. I wanted great things. Even though to some people it seemed that I was doing well, inside, a familiar feeling was creeping back into my head. This was not my life. This was not who I am supposed to be. I am not normal, and I will never be normal. Instead of feeling sad, however, I felt anger. Rage. This was not a good place for me to be emotionally. It was a dangerous place. I was in limbo, and it had to change. Change it would!

CHAPTER 19

"Ugh, I'm Mike Katz!"

It happened gradually at first. My return to the gym. It's amazing how much time one has on his hands when not dating. No wife, no family, no girlfriend, not even any hobbies. I had my job selling cars. I had moved up to a sales position at a Volkswagen/Porsche dealership. At first, that made me feel like a big deal, having my name on a business card next to the word "Porsche." The dealership was family-owned and very slick-looking. Management let me do pretty much as I pleased as long as I sold cars, which I did. Without strict guidelines and someone constantly trying to make me follow some sales script and silly procedures, I flourished. At first, this was enough to occupy my mind. However, it faded quickly, and I needed more. I needed a challenge.

I began working out again in the evenings at IRONWORKS GYM. It was not like I had completely stopped training, but I certainly had not been training seriously for some time. At first, my body felt like a beginner's. Everything hurt. After training my legs, I could not walk properly for several days.

For some reason, I enjoyed this pain. It simply made me feel ALIVE again. My body responded quite quickly, and before long, I was once again benching over 300lbs and squatting over 400. The muscle was coming back. In addition to the training, I had started dating a beautiful girl I had met at the gym by the name of Mandy. She was very stylish with a great sense of humour. We really enjoyed each other, and for the most part, we got along great. She had a son, Kyle. A very well-behaved and polite 8-year-old that was a joy to be around.

There was only one thing I made very clear right from the get-go: training was VERY important to me. It was a part of me, and it always would be. I never again wanted to watch my body get weak and have working out become something "I used to do" because of a relationship.

After a couple of months, I started getting familiar with the gym regulars and found myself training with some of them on occasion. During training one day, one of the gym regulars asked me if I was prepping for the Novice Bodybuilding Competition that was coming up in 8 weeks.

I answered, "No, I just train for fun."

His reply was to be something that would trigger something in me. "You should, man. You have the right shape, the right genetics. You would do well."

That got me thinking and remembering that at one time, I had dreams of becoming like Arnold. There was nothing holding me back now. Other than fear and self-doubt, of course, and that would have to be dealt with, not unlike walking through the doors of Pan Am Boxing Club for the first time. After all, I was no kid; I was now 35, pretty old to be STARTING to compete in bodybuilding competitions.

The other dilemma was the thought of standing on a stage flexing my muscles in front of an audience while wearing a posing suit that made Speedo's from the '70s seem large by comparison. Still, there WAS the challenge of it and the artistry of sculpting the body. That is what appealed to me on a very deep level. It was not unlike the drawings I did as a child; only now the art would be my own physique. I would be my own canvas.

The next step was telling Mandy. I was afraid she would laugh at me or think it was silly. Instead, she was supportive to a point. She asked me not to get "too big" or use steroids. I had never used steroids in my life and assured her that getting "too big" never happened overnight or by accident.

Once I had told her, I knew I had to do it. It was like a contract with myself now. I had said it out loud, so it was no longer a "maybe I might compete one day" situation. I registered for the show and paid my entrance fee.

Training to be "in shape" and training for a bodybuilding show are two very different animals I was to find out. Yes, in both endeavours you lift weights. That is pretty much where the similarities began and ended. Bodybuilding for competition can be all-encompassing.

Now you have to be concerned with how every single muscle on the human body looks. Everything has to be in balance. For example, if you have chicken legs and a massive upper body, you will definitely not do well.

You need a balanced bone structure, which you either have or you don't. The percentage of body fat has to be so low that each muscle group can be seen clearly. This is called separation. When your body fat is under 5%, you feel awful. On top of this, you will be dehydrated so that no water will obscure muscular definition. You will look your best but feel completely weak and totally exhausted. While in this state, you will be flexing every muscle at the same time during the mandatory poses as the judges compare your body to the other competitors. Until you do it, there is no way to describe how absolutely different it is from other sports. I feel it is more of an art form than a sport. You have to eat 6-7 meals a day, mainly consisting of protein, generally very low or no carbohydrates, and small amounts of healthy fats.

I knew how to train to be large and powerful. Now for the first time, I had to monitor everything I ate. I did cardio for the first time since I had started weight training. Also, I had to learn how to pose properly. All of these things were very foreign to me. It was hard giving up eating everything under the sun, and I truly hated cardio.

As far as posing, I could not have lucked into a better teacher. Rob Belisle. Rob was one of the gym regulars and was a Nationally Ranked Bodybuilder that was known for getting ridiculously ripped for contests. He looked like a walking anatomy chart. In person, it was mind-blowing to see someone that looked like that. We had often chatted in the gym and sometimes worked out a bit together. I hadn't really told anyone other than Mandy that I would be competing at Novice, so I was surprised when Rob approached me one day and asked me if I was doing the show.

I asked him, "How did you know? I keep my body covered up."

"I can see it in your face. Let's see your abs," he asked.

When I lifted my shirt, he asked me, "How many weeks out are you?"

I said, "Three."

His reply was to the point, "Want some help? You need it. You're not lean enough."

I was thrilled with his honesty and his offer. He also offered to teach me how to pose and how to perform my posing routine.

With Rob's help, I progressed more in the last three weeks than I had in the previous five. What really shocked me was how tough posing was. For some unknown reason, I thought it would be easy. How hard could it be after all? Every guy on the planet spends his youth checking out his muscles growing up.

Little did I know.

The first day we practiced posing, we met upstairs in a room that the bodybuilders used to practice posing in at IRONWORKS GYM.

"Ok, Todd, hit a front double biceps shot," Rob instructed.

Up went my arms into the pose.

He continued, "Ok, raise the arms up a bit. Squeeze them harder. Now bring in your stomach, flex your legs...."

I was starting to shake from the effort it took to contract all these muscles at once. This is how it went, on and on. Rob was analyzing and correcting.

By the time I was done with the second pose that he had taught me, I was sweating and was completely out of breath.

Rob chuckled, "Not so easy, is it?"

When I caught my breath, I stammered, "Looks easy when you do it!"

He explained that he had practiced for hours and hours over the course of many years and that posing was as important as any other aspect of preparation.

Truly, Rob made it look effortless. When he posed, he looked like a statue come to life. When I posed, I looked like a shaky schoolboy doing his best to look built.

I hung in there, working on my posing daily. Rob choreographed a simple posing routine for me as well. In a bodybuilding competition, you have to perform a one-minute posing routine to the music of your choosing. The idea is to highlight the strengths of your physique while minimizing any weak areas you might have. Rob was a master of this as well.

Slowly, I improved. It was tiring, especially while depleting your body.

Posing trunks, ah yes, the dreaded posing trunks. This was yet another aspect of competing as a bodybuilder. Obtaining and wearing "posing trunks." This was not something I was looking forward to. It was, however, a necessary evil. How else, after all, can one display the body if it is covered up? What I was to soon discover was that the trunks fellows wore in Arnold's era were positively large compared to the modern version.

In my city, there was only one store that sold these trunks. It just so happens that they mostly sold outfits for figure skaters and female dancers. Walking in there took some courage. I nervously looked around, looking obviously lost, when an elderly woman approached me. She had to be about 60 years old with a sweet face.

I started to stammer out the words, "I n-need posing trun..." when she finished the sentence for me with a chuckle and a smile.

She directed me to one solitary rack that had these little marble bags in many different colours and materials. Some were flat colours, and others were shiny. All of them looked terribly inappropriate for a 35-year-old man to be wearing.

I picked out a basic black and a basic blue and went to pay for them. The saleslady looked at me like I was nuts and said sternly, "You have to try them on!"

I tried to say that would not be necessary, and she continued, "It is very important that they fit properly. What happens if you get to the show and they are too big or worse yet, too small!?!"

"Good point," I thought.

She led me to a change room and closed the curtain behind me. I slipped on the blue ones. I looked in the mirror and was instantly mortified.

"Really?" I thought. "These are ridiculous."

It was shocking how small they were, not to mention when wearing them, there was no possible way to hide any physical flaws whatsoever. It was humbling, to say the least. Little did I know, the saleslady was waiting right outside the changeroom.

"Well, let's see," she ordered.

This was starting to seem like a bad dream. The store was full of women and girls, and I am standing there in what amounted to be nothing more than a blue handkerchief covering my ass and privates. I slowly opened the curtain but did not dare step out. I just stood there feeling very violated. This was not her first rodeo, however, and she stepped right in.

"Oh no, these won't work at all. They are way too big. Turn around." I did as I was told.

"Look here," she said, grabbing the tiny bit of material that was covering my ass. "Look how loose this is. This will never do. As you get leaner, they will get even looser. Wait, I will get you some that will fit."

I stood there trying to look composed as young girls and their mothers passed by snickering.

"Here." She thrust a pair of tiny black trunks into my hand and shut the curtain. I put them on. These black ones were way smaller. I felt the blood rush from my face as I looked at the tiny piece of material that barely covered me.

I guess I waited too long, and the curtain was opened for me.

"Ok, let's see. Ahh, yes, much better. They will be a bit small now, but in a few weeks, they will be perfect, you will see."

I meekly stuttered, "I'll take them."

I changed and brought my purchase to the front counter. I could see why they sold posing trunks. This tiny bit of material cost $50.00. As the sales lady rang them up, she looked at me and smiled.

Then she said, "Don't worry, hon, you will do just fine." She winked at me as she said it. My face was hot and red with embarrassment.

I managed a weak "thank you" and hurried out of the store. Until the day of the show, I would have repeated dreams of my trunks ripping at the seams onstage. She was right. By the time of the show, they fit perfectly.

It seemed like time was standing still those last couple of weeks. It wasn't unlike waiting for my first boxing match. I was nervous and filled with anxiety. Try to imagine standing in front of hundreds of strangers, in your underwear, tanned to an unnatural colour, covered in oil, and flexing your muscles. And just to top it off, a panel of judges are going to be judging your body. It's no wonder I was nervous.

Finally, the day of the weigh-in/registration arrived. The weigh-ins usually take place the night before the contest. In amateur contests, there are weight divisions, much like in boxing. This way, the competitors will be competing against individuals roughly the same size. I was not mentally prepared for the weigh-in at all. I did not realize how much of a mental game bodybuilding can be. It is one thing to look good and pose in front of your mirror at home. When you are by yourself with no one to compare to, you are a Mr. Universe. It is quite different being in a room full of extremely muscular, well-built individuals.

All of a sudden, you might start to realize that maybe you do not look as good as you think you did. Not to mention all the bodybuilders that are there to support their buddies, and possibly, clients. Past champions and current, looking to see what possible competition might be coming up the ranks. Girlfriends and wives as well, not to mention all the female competitors looking impossibly fit and tanned. Everyone is checking everyone else out.

I was no different, scanning the room to see who I thought I might be going up against. Each weight class is called up one by one to weigh in. I was to be in the light heavyweight class, up to 198lbs. There were eight athletes in my class. When they called up the light heavyweight class, we all had to stand up, strip down to our trunks, and get officially weighed.

Once we had all shed our tracksuits, the winner was very apparent. His name was Craig. He was much shorter than me, 5 ft 7 compared to my 6 ft.

"Fuck," was the word that came to mind when Craig took off his tracksuit. He was very thickly muscled and very lean. He was shredded, as the bodybuilding world calls it. He had more muscle than me and was more complete.

Unlike many of us, Craig had trained for a long time before he decided to enter his first show. He was leaving nothing to chance, unlike myself that had entered the last minute. Yes, I had been training just as long as Craig, perhaps longer. However, I had mostly trained as a powerlifter, and it showed. My body lacked polish and the deep cuts needed to win. What I had was a good base, structure, and balance.

Still, seeing Craig was definitely playing games with my mind. I was beaten before the contest even started. Looking at the others in my class, I felt that placing in the top five would be reasonable, and that became my goal. Once I had weighed in and officially registered and sat through the athletes' meeting, I could not get out of there fast enough.

After the weigh-ins, I went to Rob's apartment. He was going to help me put my tan on. Even though I had a good, dark tan from the sun on stage, it would never be dark enough. For many years bodybuilders had been using products such as Pro-Tan and Dream-Tan to make them as dark as possible. The reason being that under the bright stage lights having dark skin helps the muscularity to be clearly visible. If you were of a dark complexion, you had a huge advantage over pale-skinned competitors that simply looked washed out under the glaring lights. These tanning products evened the playing field.

Having your tan put on is a painstaking process. You literally stand there while someone paints you. Then you have to let it dry, then repeat the process two or three more times. After the first coat, I was darker than I had ever been in my life despite being olive-skinned. When Rob told me that I was getting two more coats, I could not believe it. "This looks weird," I said.

Rob replied, "Trust me, onstage, you will look amazing!"

Looking in the mirror, all I could see were my eyeballs and teeth.

Mandy and I had moved in together by that point in our relationship, and when I got home, her expression said it all.

"I know, I know," I said, shaking my head. "It looks weird, but apparently, onstage, it will look better."

"I hope you're right cause you to look crazy right now," she said in between fits of laughter.

I had to laugh as well. I did look crazy.

I barely slept. Before I knew it, I was at the contest that was being held at The Pantages Theatre. It is a beautiful old theatre in downtown Winnipeg. One by one, the various classes were called onstage to perform the mandatory comparisons. This is referred to as the Pre-judging. It is where the winners and different placings are decided. The evening portion of the show, or the "Finals," is more for the audience than anything. It is during the night show that you get to perform your posing routine, and the awards are handed out.

A few minutes before my class was to be called on stage, we all started pumping up with dumbbells and resistance bands as well as push-ups. Then there was the announcement, "LIGHT HEAVYWEIGHT CLASS, YOU'RE UP NEXT!"

There I was, standing in the wings in my little banana hammock, tanned and oiled up after only eight weeks of preparation. Everyone else had been prepping all year and dieting hard for 3-4 months. I was at a huge disadvantage. Not to mention, I was yet to realize just how prevalent the use of anabolic steroids and other substances was when competing as a bodybuilder.

They announced to us, "NEXT UP, THE LIGHT HEAVYWEIGHT CLASS!"

With a very deep breath, I thought to myself, "I am REALLY going to do this. Here we go!"

And just like that, after countless years of only dreaming about it, my bodybuilding career began. I do not remember much about being on stage, other than how tiring it really is to hit poses while dehydrated and nervous. It really was a no-brainer as to who was going to win.

Craig was far and away better than everyone else. Still, I WAS hoping to crack the top 5.

When I performed my individual posing routine, I remember the feeling of indifference from the audience. Bodybuilding fans are tough. They want to see an explosion of muscle and a ripped physique. Truthfully, I had neither. I had good shape with some size but was really pretty average. Eight weeks was just not enough time to get ready. I did not embarrass myself by any stretch, but I certainly did not stand out.

When they announced the top five and my name wasn't called, I simply walked downstairs to the bathrooms and started wiping off the posing oil. I found out later that I had placed 6th. I looked at myself in the mirror, and a strange feeling started to come over me. Anger. Frustration. Disappointment.

As I was looking in the mirror, a scene from the Bodybuilding Documentary "Pumping Iron" popped into my head. It was when Mike Katz had just found out he had not made the top three at the Mr. Universe in the tall men's category. He was one of the favourites to do well and is a legend in the sport. He ended up placing fourth. Mike made his way downstairs as the cameras followed him. The disappointment in his face and voice was very evident. It was very moving. You could feel his pain. I looked at myself in the mirror. What I saw looking back at me did not make me happy at all.

"Oh my God," I thought to myself. "Ugh, I'm Mike Katz!"

Right then and there, I made a decision: this was NOT going to happen again. Next year, they would know my name.

CHAPTER 20

Round Two

After feeling being destroyed in my first bodybuilding competition, I knew I needed a plan. If I was to do well at this "sport," it was going to take a lot more than eight weeks of rushed prep. It wasn't that I had any big dreams of winning the Mr. Olympia or Mr. Universe titles. However, after looking at the photos from the show, I realized that had I been in shape, aside from Craig, no one would have beaten me.

My structure and proportions were the best in the class. What I lacked was deep muscle separation, not to mention that the eight weeks of harsh dieting caused my body to go into a catabolic state. I simply started to use muscle as fuel when I cut my calories too low. Not having any steroids in my system to prevent this, I ended up looking small and smooth. My goal was to see if I was any good at this. I figured that if I prepared properly and still had my ass handed to me, well, then at least I knew. Knowing is half the battle, and I didn't want to look back later in life and wonder if I could have been any good.

Step one – talk to the head judge.

Feedback is key. Before I could put together a plan, it seemed to me that perhaps I should get the opinion of the person that knew more than anyone what the judges were looking for. The head judge for Manitoba was also the head judge for Canada. Debbie Karpenko. To look at Debbie, you would not peg her for a National Bodybuilding judge. A short, middle-aged woman of average build with a sweet smile and very pleasant disposition. She very patiently answered all of my questions. I was very careful not to debate what she told me. Rather I looked at it as an opportunity to learn where I needed to improve the most. Bodybuilders often take judges' decisions very personally. It is almost never personal, and for the most part (with a few exceptions), the judges get it right.

I took some solace in the fact that she echoed what my own thoughts were. "You have great structure and balance with pleasing lines, Todd. You need more size and much better conditioning."

At least I knew that my observations were on the right track.

Step two – talk to Rob Belisle.

Now that I knew what I needed to do to improve, it only made sense to seek out the knowledge of someone that had been there, and not only had he done it, but he had also done it very well. I called up Rob and asked if I could pick his brain.

He invited me over to his apartment to chat.

"Rob, I want to take the year to prep for novice. I need to be bigger and shredded. If you tell me what to do, I will follow it. Maybe I'm wrong, but I think genetically I was better than those guys, just needed more time."

I had an idea as to what was coming, what he was going to suggest.

"You are at a huge disadvantage when you do it without steroids. Having the year to prepare will help a lot. But you know as well as I do when you start hard dieting, you are going to lose muscle. I'm not telling you to take them. That's your call. Just telling you how it is. Ninety-nine percent of the guys you compete against will be using gear."

This was not an easy decision for me. Steroids are talked about openly now. That is a fairly recent development in the bodybuilding world. Steroid use is rampant. What was once the domain of bodybuilders, powerlifters, and elite athletes is now common practice. Teenage girls use steroids and cutting agents to lose body fat. Young guys that barely workout use them to boost aggression and build "bar muscles." They are everywhere. I realized that to be competitive, this was a bridge I had to cross.

I asked Rob if he would instruct me on how to use them if I decided to go down that road.

His answer was, "Yes, and I will make sure you do it safely."

That gave me a small amount of relief. I told him that I wanted to discuss it with Mandy, and I would let him know what my plan was.

To say I was dreading the upcoming conversation with Mandy is an understatement. I was falling in love with her, and what she thought of me mattered. I didn't want to be like so many of the guys I knew from the gym that were taking loads of steroids and lying to their wives and girlfriends about it.

I was pretty sure I was going to do it. Either way, I just did not want to lie about it. I was already gaining my muscle back now that I wasn't starving for a competition. Many people had assumed I had run juice for years. Not many guys were benching 400lbs without drugs, so I was used to the accusations. I could handle that.

So it wasn't that I was small. After all, I had been training for over 15 years. The problem was the muscle loss during contest prep. I wanted to make Mandy understand all of this, that I wasn't going to endanger myself or turn into a monster. Rather, I wanted to even the playing field.

I decided to broach the subject while we were going for a walk.

"Babe, I have decided I want to compete again next year. This time though, I want to take it seriously."

She shot a concerned look at me, "What does that mean, take it seriously? You tried your best."

I knew this was about to get rough. Mandy was not one to hide her feelings.

I continued, "Well, I will train all year, eat properly…and I am going to probably take some juice." I said the last part very quietly and quickly.

Her reaction was immediate and to the point. "WHAT?!? Are you kidding me? You're going to take steroids for this stupid contest? You promised you would never do that!!!"

It took a LOT of explaining after she lost it for a few minutes. I had to explain how steroids work, what they actually do in the body, and also that when taken in low doses and not abused, there was minimal risk to their use.

I remained very calm throughout. Mandy was a very intelligent woman, so I had to make it make sense to her in order to get her support. She eventually agreed not to kill me. I think she appreciated that I was honest about it.

There was one last thing I had to ask of her. "Babe, I will need your help. I will need you to give me the injections."

An evil smile followed by a giggle was her response. "You're going to enjoy that part, aren't you?" I asked. She just continued to smile at me in an unsettling way.

Thus, my journey down the road to my imagined bodybuilding superstardom began. Ok, no. Not really. Even though I had been around the bodybuilding scene for many years, I was always on the peripheral edge of it. I was entering into it with blinders on. I was about to learn a lot. In my mind, I was living in a lost era—the days of Arnold and Franco, Lee Haney and Joe Weider, and his magazines. Photoshoots on a beach with girls in bikinis. All of this, well, it didn't really exist anymore.

For some reason, my childhood dreams of being some kind of superman had started to resurface. I had spent my twenties not in the pursuit of my dreams or goals. That decade was lost trying to be someone I wasn't. I still didn't feel normal, but it felt good to be working towards one of my goals for a change. For the first time in many years, I felt a fire burning inside of me. Something primal. A challenge. I had lost round one, and I was not going to lose round two.

I had acquired my first little cycle of steroids. It was very simple. Sustanon (testosterone) and Dianabol (which came in pill form). Having taken my first dose, I had visions of becoming like Arnold in a month or so. After all, I was already pretty big and strong. I reasoned that the only difference between myself and the champions was the use of steroids. That thinking proved to be way off base. Don't get me wrong, the steroids worked. The degree to which they worked was much less than I had anticipated. I gained some size and strength for sure, but nothing earth-shattering. I was to learn that the dosages I was on were very low. Also, steroids increase one's capacity to train. The body can utilize protein more efficiently, and those two things enable you to get bigger and stronger. When done correctly, it is still a slow process.

I was gaining real muscle, not water. You know those guys you see in the gym that look super bloated, puffy, and huge? That's not muscle. It's water retention. It is a result of taking large amounts of steroids and essentially eating everything under the sun. When these guys diet down to compete, they end up losing 50 lbs or more. That's when you find out what your body is actually made of.

Rob was making sure that I was doing it the right way and safely.

"This time," I thought, "they are not going to know what hit them!"

A decision in my favour was not what I wanted. This time, I was going for the knockout!

CHAPTER 21

An Epiphany

A strange thing began to occur within my wee brain during the year as I was training and prepping for my assault on the bodybuilding world. I was now 36 years old, the same age as my father when he took his own life. The competition would take place a couple of months before the anniversary of his death. Perhaps it was this realization that was the impetus to start viewing the world and my own life in a different light. I had been carrying around so much rage and bitterness for years over his death and the circumstances of it.

Instead of thinking of all the negative effects that the whole unfortunate incident had brought into my life, I started to think about what my life would have been like had my father lived. Certainly, over the years, I idealized him in my mind. He became almost a mythical being.

In reality, he was a small, average man who drank to excess. He was a good man. However, he certainly had his problems. Had he lived, my sisters and I would have been exposed to his growing alcoholism and escalating fights between my parents. My mother would have left him eventually, and we would have been torn apart as a family in a different way. I would have certainly vilified my mother and would have no doubt followed in my Dad's footsteps—a cycle of depression and severe alcoholism.

His death, in its own way, caused me to find my own path. Right or wrong, it was my path, and I was not simply becoming a carbon copy of him. I had broken the cycle. It forced me to strive to become stronger both mentally and physically. Even though I am still haunted to this day by the memory of his death, it was at 36 years old that I made peace with the fact that his death was not my fault. The other consolation was the knowledge that he indirectly passed away so that I could have a better life. If nothing else, I was an individual.

The other change that occurred in my thought process was my feelings towards my mother. For years I harboured anger towards her. I was thinking more as a child than as a grown-up. At some point, as men, we all need to MTFU (man the fuck up). Essentially, quit bitching and moaning and get on with it. LIVE YOUR LIFE! The past is dead.

My mother had a very difficult situation to deal with. Now that I was in a relationship with a woman who was a mother of a young boy, I began to see and understand how challenging parenting really was. Mandy's son was a very well-behaved and personable boy. A joy to have around. Even still, parenting was tough, expensive, and could be heart-wrenching at times. Believe me, my sisters and I were no joy to be around. We fought constantly, and we each had more than our share of problems and attitudes. My mother raised THREE of us by herself. With very little money or resources and not ONCE did I ever hear her complain. We always had food in our stomachs. There were gifts on birthdays and Christmas. In her own way, she tried to talk to me at times. She encouraged my musical abilities and certainly was a big supporter of my artwork.

As often is the case, all I could see for many years were the things she was not. Never once walking a mile in her shoes, so to speak. No longer did I feel like I knew as much as I once had. Such is the arrogance of youth. As I was getting older, I felt like I really did not know anything at all, and many of the words my mother spoke during my youth now made sense. I became an idiot, and she became smarter.

I started to remember the good that she did for me. The time she bought me a football, just because I didn't have one. How she would proudly show off my artwork to my Aunts and Uncles when they visited. When I expressed an interest in learning to play the guitar, sure as shit, she made sure that on my next birthday that I received a guitar. It started to become increasingly important to me that I did something great, something different. Not just for myself, but also, I wanted my mother to feel like she raised someone that was a success. I wanted her to feel as though she was a success as well.

For some reason, I believed that succeeding in bodybuilding could help me achieve these things. No longer was I content (not that I really ever was) to be a regular guy selling cars. I wanted that Joe Weider/Arnold Schwarzenegger dream. My focus became this.

In many ways, I started to withdraw into myself, pulling away from everyone. That included Mandy and Kyle. Even though I loved them both dearly, my tunnel vision began to kick in. That kind of focus can be a great thing. Most successful people have it. The other side of the proverbial coin is that it can cause a person to forget what is truly important in life. Bodybuilding, I was to find out firsthand, can be an incredibly selfish endeavour. Many relationships do not survive when a husband or wife decides to compete. It is all-encompassing. It takes a very strong and well-balanced mind to keep what is truly important in perspective.

To compete effectively, a bodybuilder must spend ridiculous amounts of money on food, supplements, drugs, tanning, and, these days, coaching. Let's not forget the endless hours spent in the gym training, doing cardio, and posing practice. The partners or spouses are often an afterthought. Yet, the bodybuilder will want and demand total support from our partners while often ignoring their needs. As a competitor, we become drawn into a world that is only about oneself.

We expect the world to stop and take notice. To respect our mood swings, lack of energy, and often our constant need for reassurance that we are "big enough or lean enough." Our bosses and friends may try to be supportive, but as a rule, they end up giving and rarely receiving. To top it off, only a very small handful of competitors in the world make any serious money from competing—literally less than ten in the world. Competing even at the novice level is emotionally and financially costly. It's not like playing softball or recreational hockey. Essentially, we spend thousands of dollars to win a trophy in a "sport" that goes largely ignored by the general public. The average person has no idea what even happens at a bodybuilding competition.

In many regards, bodybuilding can be a beautiful life-transforming hobby that can increase self-esteem, strength, and health. However, it can also, in many ways, be cult-like. Bodybuilders and people in the industry tend to stick together and exclude those on the "outside." After all, how could "normal" people possibly understand what we go through? We feel they judge us unfairly, yet that is often what we do to them. We forget that the key to happiness in life is much more than having a good body. In fact, some of the most miserable people I have met in my life have bodies that resemble works of art! Nothing is ever good enough, and depression is commonplace. This will often push a spouse or a partner away, and the bodybuilder will then find a person in the "lifestyle" to partner with. That can end up being its own kind of nightmare, and it often seems like, in the bodybuilding community, it is hard to keep up with who is sleeping with who as relationships within the sport are beginning and ending constantly. When one relationship fails, they begin anew with someone else in the fitness landscape. I was entering a world that was like a minefield, and you could be blown up at any time!

My intentions were good. I wanted to do something great. In many ways, I could not have picked a more dysfunctional "sport" to put my energies into. I didn't realize it at the time, but my tunnel vision was going to be my downfall.

CHAPTER 22

BOOM!

The year of training went by surprisingly fast. I developed a routine that enabled me to do everything I needed to do each day. Training effectively for a bodybuilding contest while working full time and maintaining a relationship is no easy feat. Every weekend Mandy and I would cook large amounts of food that could easily be packaged, frozen, and reheated when needed. If I was lazy, I had devised a kind of protein cake or loaf that was very quick and easy to make. I could scarf one of those down in a couple of minutes in between customers if need be. Every day was kind of the same, go to work, come home and eat. Then Mandy and I would head to the gym together. She would usually do cardio as I hit the weights. She was very supportive even if she did not quite understand my need to compete and be "different."

Just before my first contest, the gym I had been training at had closed its doors and went out of business as the owner of the gym received an offer from the Canadian Postal service to lease the building. From a business standpoint, it made a lot of sense. It did, however, leave all of us bodybuilders without a home. It had been a hardcore gym, and now we were all forced across the street to more of a "fitness centre."

The equipment was very good, and the atmosphere was very stale and generic. However, with all of us being there, the energy of the place improved—most of the competitors trained there, which was great motivation for me. If I was feeling lazy, I could simply watch Rob, or Sean or Mike, or any of the guys that I knew I could one day be up against onstage to keep me hitting my workouts hard and sticking to my food plan.

As the months went by, I had made a decision to keep my body covered up. No one would be able to see how I looked. They could not analyze my strengths or weaknesses. I would not even discuss the possibility that I was competing. I was taking a page out of a former

Mr. Olympia's playbook. Dorian Yates would hide away in his dungeon of a gym in England. He would train covered up. Then when the Olympia rolled around, he would unveil his body and simply devastate all the other bodybuilders. They nicknamed him the "Shadow" because of this practice. I thought it was brilliant. I decided that the best strategy would be to catch the other competitors off guard. "Better to be underestimated," was my thinking.

Once again, Rob was helping me with not only my posing but my nutrition and, of course, the anabolic "supplementation." I had added muscle and was getting much leaner this time around as nothing was last minute. Everything was carefully planned for a full year. You can't control who shows up at a contest or how they look. The only thing I did have control over was my own physical self.

This time around, if I was going to be defeated, I would make damn sure that it would be by a person that was amazing. Not because I was ill-prepared. Rob, and of course Mandy, were really the only people that saw how my body was changing. No one else really had much of an idea as to how I looked.

Rob was always brutally honest in his critique, which helped me to stay the course. I was to find out how tough a low-carb diet could be for an extended period of time. Not only do your energy levels suffer, but your thought process can slow down, and there are definitely periods of time where you feel mentally "fuzzy" or unclear. It is harder to be patient and tolerant of others. All in all, you feel like crap even though you look your best.

One of the areas I struggled with was not eating in the middle of the night. The habit that began with my father when I was a child when he came staggering home late in the night had stayed with me my whole life. I would wake up and eat either cereal or cookies and go back to bed.

Obviously, when you are trying to get ripped for a bodybuilding competition, this is a habit that will work directly against one's progress. So instead of the cookies or cereal, I would instead have some diet pop or perhaps one teaspoon of natural peanut butter.

On two occasions, the lack of carbs and being depleted certainly caused my brain to shut down in the middle of the night. The first time this happened, I went to the fridge to take a sip of diet pop. However, for some reason, instead of the pop, I grabbed a bottle of soya sauce. I totally unscrewed the lid and took a giant swig. Let me tell you, that was one RUDE awakening. You could not pick a more drastic opposite to a diet cola than a big mouthful of soya sauce when you are carb deprived and half asleep. I sprayed it everywhere. Sputtering and coughing and wondering what the hell just happened.

Now, you would think that one would learn something from such an incident. Not I, dear readers. About a week later, I once again staggered into the kitchen in the middle of the night. This time I was craving peanut butter. In my befuddled state, I took the dish soap, poured it onto a spoon, and shoved it in my mouth. Much worse, much, MUCH worse than the soya sauce. At least soya sauce is a FOOD product. I made such a commotion that Mandy woke up and came to see what the problem was.

After laughing her ass off at me, she simply stated, "You're an idiot," and went back to bed.

As the show approached, it became apparent to the other competitors in the gym I was going to do the Novice show. No other reason to be doing endless cardio and be super tanned in February. I definitely had the feeling that they were underestimating me. They remembered the body I had the year before, and that was certainly no threat. Not to mention, I was an OLD guy, 36. How much could I improve? Being underestimated suited me just fine.

Finally, the day of the weigh-in had arrived. Rob accompanied me to supply moral support, and in case I needed any last-minute advice. When my class was called up, I was the first one to weigh in. I stripped down to my posing trunks and weighed in, then went through the line to register and get my competitor number as well as hand in my posing music.

When I returned to where Rob was sitting, he was sitting there smiling and laughing.

"What's so funny?" I asked.

He was shaking his head, "Man, you got this. That was perfect. You already won!"

I told him not to say that. "Don't jinx it, man!"

He kept chuckling as he said, "When you took off your tracksuit to weigh in, and the other guys saw you...they all took a step back. No one wanted to even stand next to you after they saw how good you look!"

He told me after that people were coming up to him and asking him what the hell did he do to me since last year, that I didn't even look like the same guy.

I was happy; things were going to plan. I was not going to be Mike Katz this time around! That being said, I would not allow myself to think that I had this contest in the bag. Bodybuilding IS subjective, after all. One never can be sure of what the judges might be looking for on any given night. Confident yes, cocky, definitely not.

Day of the show. As we waited for our class to be called onstage, most of us relaxed with our legs elevated, eating a bit, loading up on carbohydrates to fill up the muscles with glycogen. Some guys napped. There was one individual in my class that was wandering around, talking to anyone that would listen (about himself) and endlessly hitting on female competitors half his age. His name was Don, and he was a complete jackass. He had a decent upper body and not bad conditioning, but nothing to warrant his arrogant attitude.

At one point, shortly before our class was to go on, I saw my chance to get into his head. I was pretty sure that I was going to beat him. However, due to his attitude, I wanted to take him out mentally before we ever hit the stage. Just as Arnold totally could get under the skin of his opponents (as demonstrated in the docudrama Pumping Iron), I was going to do the same to Don. I had read everything available I could find on Arnold and was well versed in his methods of psyching out other competitors.

Don was posing in front of an elevator that had mirrored doors and was obviously pleased with himself. There was a glaring weak point in his physique that I was going to exploit. Don had "chicken legs." It looked as though Don had never trained his legs in his life. My upper body was better, I was leaner, but my legs grew very easily and were literally almost double the size of his. I walked over to where he was posing and stood next to him as he hit poses.

Then without uttering a word, I dropped my sweatpants and flexed my legs once. Then I looked at his reflection as he stared at my legs. I smiled, pulled my sweats up, and walked away. He spent the next several minutes doing squats in a last-ditch effort to add size to his stick legs. It was comical. He was frantically squatting away when the ONE body part you do not pump up is the legs! Once the leg muscles fill with blood, it obscures muscular definition. So, he was making his bad legs look worse. Now they were small with no definition.

Before we walked on stage and he continued to squat, I quietly whispered to him, "It might be a little too late for your legs to grow now, Don."

Once onstage, it became apparent very quickly that the audience was pulling for me. As per Rob's instructions, when the judges would call out a mandatory pose, I would let all the other guys hit their pose first. They would have to hold their pose longer, increasing the chance that they would tire and begin to shake. It also ensured that I would be the last competitor the judges looked at.

All the posing with Rob had paid off. I posed smoothly with no shaking and a smile on my face. Something was happening that I had not expected. Every time I hit my pose, the audience would let out a loud cheer. Some people were calling out my name. One of the gym regulars, Tina (a competitor herself), was yelling out TODDZILLA with every pose I hit. This was the complete opposite of my competitive experience from the year before. It felt like I was floating.

After one pose, Don leaned over to me and said, "Wow, they sure like you."

I said nothing and continued to pose and occasionally would hit an extra pose here and there. It felt natural to be onstage. Like I was home.

At the night show or finals, as it's often referred to, we got to perform our individual posing routines. I saw just how rattled Don was during his routine as I watched from the wings. Halfway through his song, he completely forgot what poses he was supposed to hit and literally stood there, doing nothing other than laughing a nervous laugh as the audience laughed at him. This is NOT the response you want from the crowd, and the judges certainly do not look favourably upon it!

Rob and I had carefully choreographed a posing routine to Lenny Kravitz's "Stillness of Heart," the key lyric that really hit me was, "I'll keep trying." It really spoke to me as I could identify with the lyrics. The response from the crowd was not like anything I expected. The previous year I could have sworn I heard crickets chirping during my routine.

This year, the people were cheering, women were shouting. It may sound silly, but at that moment, I could have cried. It was as if I finally did not feel pain. It was the strongest high I had ever felt in my life. I felt like a winner. It is one of my fondest memories that I would not trade for anything in the world.

As I sit here writing this, I am listening to "Stillness of Heart," as tears well up in my eyes. Remembering that, for one minute of my life, I felt like I mattered. As Rocky would put it, "that I wasn't just another bum from the neighborhood." My older sister Linda had made the trip to watch me compete, which meant everything to me. Her sitting there with Mandy, cheering me on. My sister that only called me "asshole" for many years, was sitting there, watching her little loser brother triumph, people shouting his name. Linda cheered for me. The girl that I loved, Mandy, proud of me. All those people from the gym that told me I couldn't do it. It's hard to even explain it all.

I won.

Shortly after I received my trophy, I was called back on stage to receive the "Best Poser" award. That means they judged my routine to be the best. In many ways, that meant more to me than the win. After the show, people were walking up to me, telling me I blew them away. That my posing routine reminded them of the classic bodybuilders, like Frank Zane and Arnold, but it was a small show. Novice. To me, it was my Mr. Universe. I made Mandy proud. I made my sister proud.

For the first time in my life, I believed I could accomplish anything. I thought the same thing as I did after my first boxing match, "I'M NOT A LOSER!"

The next day I took my trophies to the cemetery to show my Dad. I sat, and I cried as I imagined him smiling down at me. I was the same age as when he died. I began to live. Finally.

BOOM!

CHAPTER 23

"Don't feel bad if you're last."

If one really analyzes any sport enough, it is not hard to find aspects of it that may seem silly. This is especially true of bodybuilding. Even though bodybuilders train as intensely as athletes from other endeavours, we don't actually DO anything. We pose. We literally wear skimpy little posing trunks and flex our muscles while covered in oil. I think this is why many people, myself included, choose not to view it as a sport (even though the training itself is very intense).

Instead, I saw it more as an art form, sculpting one's body into something amazing—living art. After my win at the Novice competition, I realized that what I really loved was the performance aspect of displaying all that hard work for an audience that showed its appreciation for it. Hearing people voice their approval, having people cheer for you provides a high not unlike that of a drug. After experiencing success at the Novice Competition, I quickly decided to take the next step and enter the Provincial Championships. It was held twelve weeks after the Novice and is the qualifier for the National Bodybuilding Championships. The level of competition would be much higher at Provincials. I was flying so high after the Novice win that I was totally confident I would do well. Too confident.

For once, I felt like I was onto something—the right path. I have to admit; it was quite the feeling having people come up to me and tell me how they felt about my showing at the last contest. Many would ask if I was going to compete at provincials in three months, to which I would enthusiastically respond, "Of course!"

Rob met with me several times to go over how I should maintain and try to improve my condition so that I would look better at the more competitive Provincial Championships. Working towards one contest is, of course, challenging. Maintaining that shape and improving upon it is a different type of battle altogether.

There was a piece of advice that Rob gave me that I wish, in hindsight, I would have heeded.

"Do NOT get overconfident! Everyone is going to blow sunshine up your skirt because of how you looked at your last show. You need to be better to win Provincials. You CAN win that show, but the judges will be looking for you now, and they will want to see an improvement. It's a tougher show, so do not disrespect them by showing less than your best!"

I, of course, nodded in agreement. However, in reality, I was ignoring this advice and soaking up whatever adulation came my way.

In my mind, I kept thinking, "I am already in shape, hell I have three months, tons of time!"

However, there were three individuals that had a different mindset. These fellows would be the ones standing between myself and a win. There was Craig, of course. He had taken the entire year to get better for Provincials instead of jumping into it right after his first win. Then there was Ryan and Jason. Both seasoned competitors were hungry to win that overall title. Where I was coasting, these three were busting their asses to look the best that they could. I knew they would be competing and, at first, was worried about them.

Rob assured me that IF I came in my best shape, I could beat them.

What I heard was, "You will beat them." I completely ignored that IF—big mistake.

Had Rob told me that, in all likelihood, they would kick my ass, then I might have had a shot. I had ALWAYS performed my best as an athlete and in life when I was told I would fail. I would have busted my ass. Instead, I was coasting. Overconfident.

When I arrived at the weigh-in, I realized that I had made a crucial mistake. Coasting wasn't going to get you to the top spot. Upon seeing my competition, my heart sank. Ryan, Craig, and Jason all looked great. Big and ripped. All the proportion and symmetry in the world couldn't help me now. It wasn't that I looked bad or out of shape. I was very competitive with these guys.

They were simply better.

I needed razor-sharp conditioning to even think of beating them. Especially Ryan. He was big and had a nice shape and full muscles with conditioning. Jason was the sharper of the two, but Ryan's overall package was simply the best. I ended up in third place. Embarrassment best describes my feelings after the show. Mandy's family had come to watch, and even they could tell that I was simply not going to beat these guys.

I was mad at myself. "Stupid, cocky, lazy bastard!" was the thought running through my head. To punish myself further, I made sure to talk to Debbie, the head judge, for her opinion of how I looked.

She was blunt and to the point, "You handed the victory to Ryan," she said. "Had you showed up a bit leaner than you were at Novice, you could have won the whole show."

As much as those words stung, I needed to hear this from her. Nobody came up to me after the show. No one told me I should have won or that the judges were wrong or that it was "politics." The other guys were better, and I knew it.

I spent the next week fuming and quiet. Mandy gave me a wide berth as she could see that the anger I was feeling was at myself. She was pretty good that way. Understanding. I returned to training right away, with no real plan in place. Just vague thoughts of, "guess I will wait until next year."

Then an idea popped into my head out of the blue. It dawned on me that my third-place finish had qualified me to compete at the Canadian Championships that was now 11 weeks away. I could compete there. For some reason, I could not let go of the anger that I was feeling towards myself for not trying my best. Even though I knew I would discuss it with Mandy first, I had pretty much made up my mind that I was going to register to compete at the Mr. Canada competition.

Upon arriving home, I decided to discuss it with Mandy right then and there. When I told her of my plan, the look on her face was one of concern. She looked at me like I was crazy.

"I know what you're thinking," I explained. "Why would I want to compete at a much tougher show when I could only manage a third-place finish at Provincials?"

What I had to explain to her was that I could not live with how my overconfidence allowed me to be at less than my best at Provincials. I had no visions of doing well at the National Championships. My goal was to compete in my best shape. Leave nothing in the tank and be at my best. It didn't matter to me how I would place. What was of paramount importance was that I worked as hard as possible, leaving nothing to chance. My reasoning was that if I gave it my all, I would at least be able to look in the mirror, knowing I did not wimp out. If I placed poorly, or even placed last, as long as I did everything I could, well, that was something I could live with. Also, it would give me an idea of whether or not I could hang with the serious bodybuilders, the elite in Canada.

Very few male competitors from Winnipeg ventured onto the National stage, preferring to remain big fish in a small pond and often competing year after year at the Provincial level. My goal, after all, was to see if I could make it in bodybuilding. If I got destroyed at the National level looking my best, then at least I would have peace of mind knowing that I went for it. If genetically I could not cut it, well then, I would end this little experiment and move on.

After explaining this all to Mandy, she was on board. I think she figured, "Let him get it out of his system so we can move on with our lives."

My training took on a sense of urgency again. Deciding it was best not to tell anyone that I was competing at Nationals, I kept my body covered up as I trained. I simply did not want to hear the negative thoughts of others. To most individuals in the local scene, a National show was where the monsters competed, and I knew that I would be told over and over how I was going to get destroyed there.

I had my blinders on, even though I realized that there was a very good chance that I was going to get my ass handed to me at this show, I did not want to think of it in those terms. I visualized myself as a machine, ripped and hard, polished and ready.

The same anxiety and nervousness I had always felt when prepping for a fight was present, and I utilized those feelings to push myself harder in and out of the gym. My food was spot on—no more cheating on my diet. Knowing I would not be one of the bigger bodybuilders, my goal became one of perfection. Balance and symmetry with great conditioning will always stand out on stage. I worked hard to add muscle in the right places (shoulders, back, and calves) and even harder at getting as ripped as possible. The tunnel vision was kicking in, and everything else in my life seemed to lose importance.

Everything was going to plan. I was getting ripped, progressing, and improving with no one in the gym being the wiser. Until Henry. Henry…how do I describe BIG Henry? Which is pretty much what we all called him. Picture the THING from the Fantastic Four but as a human—big, strong, thick all over, and scary. I had known Henry from Ironworks Gym. He was one of the regulars.

He started as I did, in powerlifting, later switching over to bodybuilding. He had won the Provincial Championship years earlier as I watched in awe from the audience. His physique was not a pretty one, but you could not dispute the amount of muscle he carried, and when he competed, he always showed up shredded to the bone. Henry had done well at Nationals and knew the bodybuilding game well.

As big and intimidating as he was, he was kind and patient. No matter what question I asked him in the gym, he would take the time to answer. He was well-liked by everyone. Mandy thought he was hilarious and loved him as he always treated her so kindly and not unlike a little sister. She always referred to him as "Henri (spoken with a funny French accent)."

As friendly as he was, I NEVER wanted to see him angry at me. I often imagined that if I ever had to fight him (a terrifying thought), that even if I hit him with my best shot, number one, I am pretty sure I would break my hand on his huge head. Number two…he would probably just smile and rip my arm off at the socket and bring it home for his dogs to chew on. Henry had no filter. If he thought it, he would have zero problems saying it. I used to laugh my ass off at his lack of giving a shit about what anyone thought about him. The gym we trained at was a big one.

If Henry spotted me across the room, and I shouted a greeting and asked him, "Hey Henry, how you doing?" He would invariably shout back at me in his deep gravelly voice, not only how he was doing, but he often he would list off what steroids he was currently taking.

It usually would go something like this, "Hey Henry, how's it going?"

To which he might reply (very loudly), "Good brother, I just started my tren and gh, I'm switching over to test prop and maybe thinking about adding something else!"

That would always crack up any of the regular guys, the bodybuilders, and mortify the "regular folks" that made up a large portion of the gym population. Henry knew who he was and simply did not care if you liked it or not. I really admired that about him.

It was Henry who figured out I was going to compete at Nationals. We were both at the dumbbell rack one day when I could feel his gaze upon me out of the corner of my eye.

Then he said it, loudly, "You're doing Nationals, hey?"

I froze instantly, "What? No, Henry, I'm not."

I was facing him now. He was squinting at me with that look only Henry could give.

He was very rugged-looking and could look right through you. "Why is your face all sunken in? You have contest face."

Trying to think fast, I stammered out, "I'm just staying in shape for the summer."

He continued to glare at me as I felt increasingly like a kid caught stealing in a candy store. "Bullshit Todd! You're doing Nationals, so don't lie to me!"

I sighed, "Ok, yes, Henry, keep it down. I don't want anyone to know!"

Henry laughed his big laugh, "I knew it, staying lean for summer. What crap! Want some advice?"

"Absolutely!" was my immediate reply.

"Make sure you're shredded. You look good, Todd, but you gotta be ripped and dry. You have a good physique, but it won't matter if you are smooth. Oh yeah, and don't feel bad if you're last."

I laughed, "Last place is not my goal. Thanks a lot, asswipe!" We both laughed.

"You have to understand, Todd, this is your first Nationals. There are guys that have been competing at that show for ten years trying to turn pro. The judges haven't seen you. I have seen guys that looked great get completely ignored and overlooked. Sometimes you just have to pay your dues. So don't feel bad if you're last. You look great, though, even covered up, I can see you are gonna be in shape this time!"

It WAS good advice. Honest advice. I had a new goal in addition to being in my best shape. DON'T BE LAST!!!

CHAPTER 24

"This was a mistake!"

I stood there awestruck. To say I was not prepared for what I was now looking at is a grand understatement. The weigh-in for the Canadian Bodybuilding Championships looked like an insane circus of muscle. A great deal of the FEMALE competitors are bigger and more ripped than the men at the Provincial level in Manitoba. Easily there had to be over 200 people milling about: competitors, coaches, sponsors, pro bodybuilders, and press. Later I was to find out this was the largest athlete field in the history of the Canadian Championships.

"Great timing, douchebag!" was the thought that ran through my mind upon hearing that bit of info. The mind games of being there is hard to describe. Bodybuilders I had only seen in magazines or in ads for various supplement companies were walking around. It seemed like the level of development wasn't human. Not just on the pros, on EVERYONE!

It seemed like everyone was aware of each other. They all knew one another. I was catching little bits of conversation here and there.

"Have you seen Fuoad? He's going to win it!"

"I'm not sure, Mboya looks great, and Leon is here. He's a freak as well."

Some of the women had voices deeper than mine, and on some of them, you could see what looked to be stubble on their faces.

I remember thinking, "So THIS is bodybuilding." The bodybuilders appeared to be keenly aware of the mental warfare aspect of the goings-on of the whole crazy scene. If someone had amazing legs, rest assured they were in shorts. Great arms, in a tank top.

As I gazed around the melee of muscledom, one thought kept running through my carb-depleted little brain, "Don't feel bad if you're last, Todd." It was Henry's voice, of course. When my class stripped down to officially weigh-in, I realized that not placing last was going to be a tall order indeed. I took solace in the fact that I had one teammate from Manitoba in my class, Derek Robertson, a former Light Heavyweight Provincial Champion. He looked great, super shredded.

His expression told me that perhaps he was having the same thoughts as I was. Something like, "Um, maybe we should have stayed in Winnipeg!" Mboya Edwards, one of the favourites to win the show, was in our group, as well as a human cinder block named Trent Walsh, who appeared to be as wide as he was tall. Another familiar face that stood out was Trevor Martin, a former Manitoba Champion that was now competing out of Alberta. He used to train at IRONWORKS, and I remember watching him in awe as he trained. Now, I would be standing next to him onstage.

"This was a mistake! Coming here. What was I thinking? I am going to get destroyed. Maybe I should leave. Who would know?" my mind was racing with fearful thoughts.

"You would know." It was Coach K's voice in my head now, "Shoulder down."

I steadied myself and decided what the hell, it's a bodybuilding contest. I had been through much worse. When I stepped on the scale to weigh in, I was greeted with an unwanted surprise; I was 2 lbs over the weight limit for my class. The official instructed me of my two options, I could move up to the heavyweight class, or I could try and weigh in again in 30 minutes. I knew that at this point, I was definitely not big enough to be a heavyweight, so I took the second option, losing 2 lbs in 30 minutes.

The day before you compete, you are truly exhausted. Depleted, and more than likely, you are cutting water at this point, so you are dehydrated as well. Now on top of all this, I had to try and lose another two pounds. It was time for a gut check. I put on as much clothing as I could, found a staircase, and began running stairs. I would also run to the bathroom if I felt that I could urinate even a little bit.

As I stood there trying to go, I would spit out as much as I could. I felt like puking and tried to make that happen to no avail. Back to the stairs, up and down, sweating and feeling like collapsing. It was the worst 30 minutes of cardio I had ever performed in my life. When I had less than two minutes of time left, I ran back to the weigh-in area and waited my turn to get back on the scale. I kept all the clothing on until the last possible second.

Before I stepped on, I exhaled all the air out of my lungs. The official joked, "Think light thoughts." She read out my weight, "197.9lbs, Todd Payette, Light Heavyweight!" I jumped off the scale immediately. I wasn't taking any chances. I looked to my left, and the official was Debbie Karpenko, the head judge from Winnipeg.

She smiled at me with her kind eyes and quietly said, "Good work, Todd!" It was great to hear her words of encouragement at that point.

I met Mandy after the weigh-in to head back to our hotel room to begin the process of carbing up. After completely depleting the muscles, a proper carbohydrate load can refill the muscles with glycogen, essentially pumping them up and making you appear larger on stage. It's a really tricky balancing act. If you eat too many or the wrong type of carbs for your system, you can "spill over," which is a bodybuilding term that means you lost definition and look smooth. My plan was to carb up on a burger and some fries as well as snack through the night when I felt the need. At first, this feels great. After all, eating a burger and fries is fantastic after months of depleting the body. However, you can't drink any water at this point. So, after a few bites of my burger and fries, I realized that this, too, would be a challenge.

After we finished eating, it was back to the hotel room for what amounted to be a long night. This contest would be the first time that I was to try using diuretics. The list of things "I would never do" was getting shorter the more involved with bodybuilding I became. At one time in my life, I would proudly declare, "I would NEVER use steroids or drugs!" Then, of course, that changed. Then it became, "I will never use diuretics!" There had been cases of people dying from improper use of diuretics. Well, life has a way of making a liar out of us all at one time or another. I didn't know it yet, but I had just scratched the surface of what drug use in the "sport" of bodybuilding could be. I was amazed at how much a little pill could make someone with very little water left in their system pee. I spent the night waking up and going at least once or twice an hour. Sometimes I would eat a little as well after these bathroom breaks. Each time I would eat, I would quickly regret it as the food only made me want to drink water. I had never experienced thirst like this before. It was a bit scary, feeling this dry, and yet I kept going. I became convinced that by morning I would be urinating out dust or perhaps sand!

Christmas morning! That's what it felt like when I woke up. After a long night of being ridiculously thirsty, peeing, and eating, I could finally see if that damn little pill made a difference. I felt exhausted. I walked over to the full-length mirror in our room and flexed my legs.

"What the hell!?" I could not believe what I was seeing. I rubbed my eyes and flexed my quads again. "Hollllyyyyy shiiiiiiit!" It was as if I had grown a new set of legs overnight! There were deep cuts and striations in my legs that I had never seen before.

I had to wake up Mandy. Maybe I was imagining this. I led Mandy over to the mirror and instructed her, "Ok, now watch my quads when I flex." I hit a leg shot, and her eyes grew wide. "Fuuuuck," was all that came out of her mouth.

"It's crazy, right?" I asked. She asked me to do it again, and I flexed hard.

"Your legs never looked like that before," she said, shaking her head. I could not get over it. There was a very noticeable difference after the body rids itself of so much water. In order for this to work at all, you must already be very lean. Once your body fat percentage is very low, the only thing that usually obscures muscular definition is water. It was remarkable. No longer did I care that I was thirsty. This was the best I had ever looked for a contest.

I ate a big breakfast consisting of pancakes, bacon, and eggs, with again, no water. From there, it was time to head to the venue. The show was very well organized. There was a small fitness expo with various booths set up with all of the latest in everything bodybuilding-related. Each weight class had its own dressing room where we pretty much just sprawled out and relaxed until it was time to pump up.

They had set up a separate area filled with weights for us to use before hitting the stage. As we relaxed in our dressing room, I noticed that the heavy hitters of our class were not present. Trent, Trevor, and Mboya were nowhere to be found. That suited me fine as the three of them certainly did not make me feel like my chances of success were very high. At one point, three of the guys got up and were all hitting leg poses in the mirror. I watched from my corner of the room.

I thought, "Hmmm, I don't think any of those three guys have legs better than mine." I decided to have an "Arnold" moment. I walked up to the three of them, positioned myself right in the middle and dropped my sweats, and hit a leg pose. I flexed very hard as every muscle in my quads contorted and snapped to attention. I said nothing, pulled up my sweats, and went back to my corner.

I could hear one of the guys quietly say, "Did you see his quads? Holy shit, that's crazy!"

I smiled. Maybe I wouldn't be in last place after all.

It was finally time to hit the stage. I remember waiting in the wings nervously just before we were to walk out. The cheers and response from the audience seemed very loud. I peeked around the corner so I could see the crowd. I felt a lump in my throat as I realized that there were easily four times as many people at this show as my previous three shows had in attendance combined.

"Welcome to the big leagues," I thought as a wave of anxiety washed over my whole body.

The light-heavyweight class was a large class. They had half of us go through the mandatory poses at a time. Then we all returned to the back of the stage, and they started calling out competitor numbers for more comparisons. This would be the top five. The first one called out was Mboya. No surprise there. Then a fellow named Farzad Ghotbi—he looked great. Then it was Trevor and Trent, and then I heard them announce, "Number 101, please."

No one moved. They called it again. I remember thinking, "Who is 101? Wait a minute, that's me!"

I took my place in the top five lineup. I could feel myself smiling. I heard Mandy screaming to my right. I looked over. I could just make her out. Her expression was priceless. She looked like she was beaming! Debbie started calling out the mandatory poses. I was careful in each one, setting them up, transitioning smoothly. Smiling.

They kept moving us around, carefully looking us over. They ran us through the poses three times. I was exhausted. I had never been in a comparison this long before. As much as I was tired, thirsty, and hot, I did not care. I was in the top five at the Mr. Canada!

The crowd response was fantastic. Over everyone, I could hear Mandy. I was so happy she was there to share this moment with me. It had always seemed that I had competed alone in sports as a youth, with no parents or family coming to watch. It felt incredible. Finally, the judges dismissed our group from the stage. I bowed to the judging panel and picked out Debbie's face, making eye contact with her as I mouthed the words thank you to the judges.

At a National event, only the top five in each class get to perform their posing routines as there are simply so many competitors there is no way that they could fit everyone in. I waited backstage as they announced the light heavyweight class. The entire class then went out as the judges ran us all through our mandatories one more time. Then they called out the top five.

All I can remember is hearing, "From Manitoba, Todd Payette!"

Mandy was screaming and cheering as I walked back out onstage.

They put us through our poses again. Then it was time for our individual routines. It seemed like a dream. I performed my routine from novice and received a nice round of applause from the audience. I walked off stage, or rather floated offstage, and waited for them to announce the top three.

"Fifth place," I thought, "right on, yup, that's not last place, not last place at all!"

The top three were of no big shock. Trevor was third, Trent second, and Mboya winning it. Mandy and I had planned to meet at the fitness expo, so I changed and headed over there.

On the way there, I heard my name called out, "Todd, wait up!"

It was Mike Mckee. He was the Vice President of our provincial federation. Mike came over to me. "Todd, way to go! That was amazing!"

"Thanks, Mike, fifth place! Man, I can't believe it."

Then Mike said something I really didn't expect, "Todd, you weren't fifth. You were fourth!"

I couldn't believe it. I challenged him on it, "Mike, don't bullshit me, there's no way."

Mike was shaking his head, "Todd, I saw the scorecard. You're fourth. We are all proud of you!"

I gave Mike a huge hug. Mike was a bear of a man and loved by all of us that competed in Manitoba. It was great getting such good news from someone I respected so much!

I went to find Mandy. I felt like Rocky at the end of the movie when he went the distance, and all he cared about was finding Adrienne. People kept stopping me and shaking my hand, telling me congratulations, and asking me questions.

All I wanted to do was find Mandy. Finally, I saw her. As we embraced, I whispered into her ear, "Fourth place, could not have done it without you, I love you!" She had tears in her eyes. I knew right then and there that I wanted to marry her.

I was not just another bum from Elmwood. I was not a loser. I had ventured out of my little pond and swam with the sharks and did not get eaten. I thought of my Dad, then of my Mom. I wanted her to be proud.

After all, I was not last place!!!

CHAPTER 25

The Universe and Beyond

Shock. That probably best describes the feeling I was experiencing after my fourth place finish at the Canadian Bodybuilding Championships. After all, my goal was to not finish in last place. Nothing had prepared me for success. In some ways, I was on top of the world. Looking back, it was the beginning of the end. Not knowing how to process success, I would begin a long slow spiral down into my own personal hell. For now, however, I sat in the passenger seat during the long drive home, smiling and thinking, "Fourth in the country, wow."

Mandy was happy for me. Her parents were happy for me. I assumed that my Mom would be happy for me as well. Even at 36 years of age, I still wanted to make her proud of me. We did not talk very often, but I figured that this success warranted a phone call to her.

After making some small talk, I decided to fill her in on what I felt was a great moment in my life.

"Hey Mom, so I just competed in another bodybuilding competition. It was the MR. CANADA!"

"Oh really?" was her reply.

"Yeah! It went really well…."

"Did you win?" she interrupted. I felt some of the wind leave my sails,

"Um, no, I placed fourth!" An uncomfortable silence followed for a few seconds.

"Do you win money for fourth place?"

I sighed and felt myself get smaller, "Mom, it's a prestige thing, like an honour. It means that out of all the thousands of guys that compete in my class in Canada, I was fourth!"

More silence and then, "Oh, that's nice."

It felt like a blow to the gut. After that, I quickly wrapped up the conversation and sat there stunned.

Then I got angry. My mind raced with thoughts like, "What does she know? Seriously, she never accomplished anything great. Who does she think she is? She was a waitress her whole adult life and then married a man with money. Now she acts like she's a big deal. I don't need her approval. Screw it. I don't need anyone!"

Of course, all these thoughts were because I was hurt. I thought that she would be proud of me. Looking back, I realize that she had no way to comprehend what fourth place at the Mr. Canada contest meant. How much work it took, the sacrifice! There was also no way for her to understand what it meant to me on an emotional level. For her, success equaled money, and money equaled success. She could not relate. It was not her fault. At the time, it cut me deeply.

One of the very real emotions that many competitors experience after a competition is one of sadness. You no longer have an immediate goal. Everything you have been doing for many months has been directed towards a competition. Once it's over, a huge dark cloud can descend over you as you think, "Now what?" For me, I had a new goal. Turning pro. That was a year away. In my mind, I felt that fourth place at my first Nationals meant that not only could I swim with the big sharks, but I could also succeed at that level. So even though I felt a little lost for a few weeks, I started turning my attention towards returning the next year and winning.

I started to taste a tiny bit of success. Garry Bartlett from MuscleMag International Magazine mentioned me in his coverage of the show. It was only one sentence, but I was thrilled. Musclemag was my favorite bodybuilding publication which I had been reading for years, and now my name was in it!

Self-promotion is very important in the physique world, so I set about the business of getting my name out there. I sent several pictures from a photoshoot that I had booked, as well as contest pics, to several (too many to count) supplement companies in the hopes that one of them might think my look, which was a very "traditional" one, might appeal to at least one of them. I never for a minute thought that I would get signed by the company that eventually took a chance on me.

Muscletech was one of the largest supplement companies in North America at the time. After seeing my photos, they called me and offered to fly me down to Toronto. They paid for everything, flights, hotel, and food. I still remember pulling up to their office building. It was very impressive and modern. As I got closer to the entrance, I saw a van parked out front with young fellows unloading various types of training equipment. As I neared them, one of the young guys was about to lift a massive dumbbell that looked to weigh about 140-150lbs.

He was a thinly built young man, and I asked him, "Hey bud, you want a hand with that?"

He looked at me and laughed and proceeded to lift it with one hand quite easily and set it down. He only looked like he weighed maybe 150lbs himself. Standing there with my jaw dropped open, he looked at me and said, "Go ahead, lift it!"

With a look of confusion on my face, I bent over and picked up the very heavy-looking dumbbell. With shocking ease, I lifted it off the ground.

"It's a prop dumbbell. It weighs maybe 50-60 lbs.," he explained. "It weighs just enough to make the muscles do a bit of work. That way, in photoshoots, it still looks like the model is straining."

I laughed, "That's hilarious!" That's how guys in contest shape still manage to lift these huge weights for photoshoots even when they are weak and depleted. I was quickly learning that not everything in bodybuilding was as it seemed!

Inside of the Muscletech offices, it was even more impressive. Instead of vending machines filled with soft drinks, they were filled with protein and energy drinks. I was brought to the in-house fitness centre, which was better equipped than most large commercial gyms. There were lights set up, and a photoshoot was taking place.

After the tour, I was invited to have lunch in the cafeteria. Without a doubt, it was the best cafeteria I had ever seen! It was like it was set up especially for bodybuilders. There was a chef that was cooking chicken breasts and vegetables along with rice. The vending machines with protein drinks were there as well, along with other ones stocked full of protein bars. Most of the staff looked in great shape. This was a company that took an interest in the health of its employees.

After lunch, I sat down with one of the athlete reps to go over what they were offering me. It was their standard package they offered to amateurs. It was a contract spanning two years. They wanted me to compete at Nationals again and would provide me with $1000.00 worth of supplements every month in addition to covering all of my costs that I incurred at the show: travel, hotel, tanning, food, and entrance fees were all to be paid for by Muscletech. If I turned pro while under contract, they would pay me an additional $2000.00/month.

All in all, it was a pretty good deal. I signed right then and there. It wasn't like I had tons of companies beating down my door to sign me. It is very difficult to get ANY sponsorship deal; being signed by one of the biggest supplement companies around sounded pretty good to me. Before I left, the athlete rep made sure to load up a Muscletech gym bag with protein drinks and other supplements to send along with me.

As I sat in the fancy hotel room that was paid for by Muscletech, I could not help but think about my "Mike Katz" moment after my first show, how the other competitors had taken me so lightly, disregarding me as a threat on any level. Now I had placed well at my first National Show. I was under contract with a major player in the bodybuilding world. I had only competed in four contests at that point in my career, and two of those had been Novice shows.

All of it left me shaking my head in disbelief. I had no skill set that had prepared me for any of it. I was being drawn into the vortex of the bodybuilding world. It's a crazy sport/business, and thousands of people participate and compete in it. Many with dreams of "making it big." It's really absurd. Unlike other professional sports, bodybuilding requires more of a mental and physical price to pay with very little chance of any substantial financial return. We pour our hearts and souls into bodybuilding. We give up food, a social life, careers, relationships and risk our health all for the glory of standing on stage for a few minutes and hopefully hearing some applause. If we are lucky enough to win, we get to take home a trophy that really is worth nothing.

When all is said and done, the bodybuilder will have literally spent thousands of dollars on food and drugs to possibly win that little trophy. Even though it made no sense on many levels, I bought into Joe Weider's bodybuilding fantasy and was ready to do anything to be the next "Arnold." What I really needed was guidance. I was flying by the seat of my pants. I had no idea what I was doing or what I was getting myself into!

It's funny looking back. In fact, if you would have told me a year earlier what was about to happen, I would have thought you were crazy. As the old saying goes, "Sometimes it's better to be lucky than good."

What happened next was a great example of that old adage coming to fruition. I had never been a big computer guy, but the reality of the internet as a tool for self-promotion was not lost on me. I had several photos posted on various sites, Facebook as well as some of the bodybuilding forums. It was because of these photos that I received an invite to compete in a regional show in the UK.

One of the organizers of this show (which would have been comparable to one of our Provincial level shows) and I had struck up a conversation about bodybuilding and the direction in which it was heading. We both felt that being huge for the sake of being huge was not only the wrong direction, but also it was dangerous as the athletes were being forced to use more and more drugs at insane levels to reach the size needed to be competitive.

This official (sadly, I can't remember his name) felt that reasonable size with balance and separation was a better way to go. The "Arnold" era was a great example of that physical ideal. Since he believed my physique represented that look, he extended an invite for me to come over and compete in his show.

I thanked him and then took a huge chance and decided, "What the hell, let's roll the dice!"

I knew that the federation that he represented (NABBA), which was the oldest bodybuilding federation in existence, also held the very prestigious MR. UNIVERSE contest. After thanking him, I made him a counteroffer, "Thank you very much for the invite to your show. However, I am currently ranked fourth in Canada as a Light Heavyweight, so my focus is competing in higher level contests at this time." I continued, "IF you extended an invitation to compete in the amateur division of the MR. UNIVERSE Contest I would be honoured to attend and compete."

Realistically, I expected a polite brush-off. Instead, I received a reply I truly did not expect, "I think that's a great idea. Let me forward that idea to Val Charles."

At this point, I thought, "Well, that's the end of that."

Two weeks later, I received an email with an official invitation to compete in the Amateur Division of the MR. UNIVERSE Contest. I re-read that email probably ten times over.

While the Mr. Olympia is regarded as the highest bodybuilding title that one can win, The Mr. Universe has the longest history and is more recognized by the general public at large. The title alone, "MR.

UNIVERSE," conjures up an almost mythical vision of someone with classic and god-like proportions. At one time, the Mr. Universe was THE top title in the world, and previous winners include every major bodybuilding legend in existence, from Steve Reeves to Arnold. Even Sean Connery once competed in this great contest! Being a student of the history and much preferring the "look" of the past, MR. UNIVERSE winners, I was on cloud nine. The Universe had long been a dream of mine. To even stand on the same stage that all my heroes once graced was my personal Mount Everest!

The local news stations picked up on the story, "Winnipeg man invited to the Mr. Universe."

My ex-girlfriend Lisa even invited me to be on her morning radio program. We had a lot of fun with that one. I started off the interview doing my best ever "Arnold" impression without first warning her or her co-host. They burst into laughter, and we had a great time with it!

Our local magazine "STYLE" did a full two-page story on me as well, also written by Lisa. Of course, with any level of success, you may achieve, there will always be some individuals that seem to get agitated at your "luck."

Slowly I was made aware of some folks in the local bodybuilding community that did not like the attention I was getting. "Why did Todd get signed by Muscletech? The Universe? How did that happen?" and so it went. I wish it didn't bother me, but it did. What people did not see or know about was all I was doing behind the scenes trying to market myself. I could not even count the number of people I reached out to. I was doing what I thought Arnold would do, albeit on a much smaller scale. I would forge ahead, hell-bent on my goals, and pushing everything else to the side. After all, I was going to the Universe and beyond!!!

CHAPTER 26

Highway to Hell

It's hard for me to explain what was driving me at that point in my life. Why was it so important for me to be different? Bodybuilding was an odd choice for someone that wanted to be recognized by the public at large as a success. The average person does not understand bodybuilding or even know who the champions of the sport are. For most, it begins and ends with Arnold. Perhaps it was the physicality of it, the challenge of one's willpower. You have to deny yourself so many things. Push your body to places that, physiologically, it does not want to go. It was an impossible endeavour in so many ways, and it demanded 100% focus not just in the gym but around the clock. For the next year, I would punish myself.

There were some joys in my life as well. I bought an engagement ring and proposed to Mandy. I took her to a quiet spot that we had visited on our very first date. I parked the car overlooking the Red River. I told her how much she meant to me. That I wanted to be a better man because of her, that I loved her and would be honoured if she would be my wife. She cried and said yes. She later admitted that when I showed her the ring that she effectively stopped hearing any of the words coming out of my mouth, and luckily, she said yes at the right moment. She called her parents immediately, and they were happy about our engagement. At that moment, I, too, was happy. Why wouldn't I be? Mandy was a beautiful, intelligent woman. Her son Kyle was a great kid. Even though I was happy on some levels, I was still fighting my personal demons. There was still the matter of doing something "different." I needed to be a success, even if it was not in the traditional sense.

My training took on an urgency. If I was going to compete in the Mr. Universe, then I would do so at my best! Mandy was thrilled at the idea of taking a trip to England, where the Mr. Universe is held. We decided to wait until after the Universe to get married as there was no way we could afford to take a trip to England and a wedding in the same year. That was assuming that Muscletech was going to be covering most of the expenses for that show.

Still, it would mean time off of work, and Mandy's expenses would not be covered, only mine. We had also planned on getting there a week early, so we had time to make sure I had the proper food, a gym to go to, and there were no last-minute surprises. Then after the contest, we could always stay for a few days and enjoy the country. Of course, I was about to find out that things do not always go according to plan.

I was already several months into my training when I decided that I better start making arrangements with Muscletech for the trip to England. I expected them to be thrilled that I was going to be competing in the Mr. Universe.

"What do you mean I would be voiding my contract by competing in the Universe?" I could not believe what I was hearing.

"Muscletech does not currently have products in the UK, so it is of no benefit for you to compete there. We want you to compete at the Canadian Championships. You can, of course, do what you want. However, if you decide to compete in the Universe, we will be cancelling your contract."

I was stunned. I was faced with a very tough decision here. After talking it over with Mandy, we decided that England would just be too expensive. Not to mention that if I won at Nationals, then that extra $2000.00/month Muscletech would pay me would be a big help to us financially.

Since the shows were roughly at the same time, I would just keep prepping as I had been. It was a heartbreaking decision for me. At the time, I felt it was the smart way to go. My hopes were that I would have another chance at the Universe if I continued to compete successfully.

This also freed us up to make plans to get married which we would do after Nationals. We decided to have a destination wedding in Mexico. That could be planned later. Right now, it was full steam ahead with my training. Other things in life mattered less to me now. Even though we were now engaged, my priority became the gym.

At work, I was really just going through the motions. My tunnel vision was becoming worse. I was slipping away from all that was important. I had increased my use of anabolic steroids and was now including drugs that would help the body shed fat.

I was now taking my body to a place it had not yet been. It was my goal to come into the show better and leaner than I was the previous year and as ripped as possible. I stuck to my diet 100%. This, of course, caused me to be exhausted all of the time. My patience was at an all-time low. I remember having to leave the dinner table and go eat by myself because I could not handle the sound of Kyle eating.

That is often the reality of taking your body to extremes. Extreme fatigue with the added bonus of increased testosterone can do bad things to your mind. Everyone has heard the tired "roid rage" clichés. The reality is, if you're an asshole, you will be a bigger asshole on steroids. For the most part, I am a very easy-going person.

Over the years, I had to learn to control my temper. There were times that it definitely got the better of me. One time in particular that comes to mind was during the prep for that show (2007 Mr. Canada). Mandy and I lived in an apartment complex that had balconies that overlooked the parking lot for the tenants. Beside that was an in-ground pool and pool house.

One summer evening, I heard several loud drunken voices coming from the parking lot. I headed out to our balcony to check it out. There was a group of young men, quite drunk and loud, on one of the balconies and another in the parking lot. They were throwing a football back and forth and making quite the racket, essentially disturbing the quiet of the whole complex.

Mandy joined me on the balcony. I have zero tolerance for drunks, and Mandy knew it. I was getting madder by the second as I am watching the football landing closer and closer to the parked cars. Closer and closer to mine. They were throwing from the second floor. The ball could easily put a dent in a car from that height.

Mandy could read me very well, "Leave it, Todd, it's not worth it."

I growled, "If that ball hits my car, they are all going to be sorry!"

Sure enough, not a minute later, the ball slams into the car parked next to mine. That was it! Close enough for me.

At this point, I am close to contest shape, nothing but muscle, and quite crazy looking. I head down to the parking lot and stride towards the young man.

"YOU THROW THAT FUCKING BALL ONE MORE TIME, AND YOU'RE GOING TO THE FUCKING HOSPITAL!"

The young man turned towards me. His eyes got wide with fear.

Then I turned my attention to the group on the balcony, "CMON DOWN IF YOU WANT YOUR ASS KICKED!" I was livid. I totally called them out, telling them they had no respect for others' property, not to mention that no one wanted to spend their evening listening to them yelling and carrying on. I then demanded an apology from them. They complied.

At that point, I did not care how many of them there were. I wanted to rip them apart. I must have looked like a rabid Rottweiler to them. They wanted no part of it, and they quieted down. As I headed back to our apartment, one of our elderly neighbours stopped me and thanked me for shutting them up. I apologized to her for using vulgar language and making a scene.

Her reply was, "It's ok dear, it worked, thank you."

When I got back to our apartment, Mandy looked at me and, while shaking her head, said, "You're crazy. You know that, right?" I just smiled and nodded.

Finally, it was time to compete. I had put every ounce of myself into my prep for this show. I was leaner than I had ever been and truly felt like death. In my mind, winning would be worth it. When I arrived for the show, there were two familiar faces at the weigh-in that would be in my class—Craig, who had destroyed me in my first show, and Rob, my mentor. I was honoured to compete against him.

When we stripped down, I could see that Craig looked amazing. Rob was not his usual shredded to the bone self.

He looked ok, but I figured, "Wow, I am going to beat Rob."

I think he thought the same thing, as he told me that I looked amazing, the best he had seen me. Rob wasn't one to hand out compliments. I walked onstage feeling very confident. Then something happened that I did NOT expect. I was not in the top five callouts for comparisons. I was in shock. How could this be? Last year I was fourth, and I was in much better shape this year. Not even top five? I was stunned. When the dust settled, Craig placed 5th, Rob 6th (I think mostly by reputation), and I placed 10th.

It made ZERO sense to me. I was expecting the top three, at least. I was one of the best conditioned in the class, with probably the best overall shape. What I did not see was this: being six feet tall, I was much taller than all the other light heavyweights. They were on average 5ft 7 to 5ft 8. Short, thickly muscled guys. It was a case of apples and oranges. My look was very different than all of them. I would have been better off to have sat out the year and gained 8-10lbs of muscle, and competed as a heavyweight as I was too tall to be a light heavyweight.

Bodybuilding is very subjective. The winners are a matter of opinion and taste. I can process this now, in hindsight. At the time, I was devastated. All these people, Muscletech, all had big expectations for me. I had failed. I was miserable and lost. I had done my absolute best and had my ass handed to me. Craig beating me again did not feel great either.

When Mandy and I got home, I did not know what to do with myself. I figured I am done. Tenth place? There was no way. What bullshit. Doesn't symmetry and proportion count for anything? The judges rewarded short blocky guys with thick guts. Yup, I was feeling sorry for myself. I spent the next five days doing nothing but gorging myself on food. Pop-Tarts, cereal, bread, pizza, burgers, you name it, I ate it. I gained 38lbs in five days. For the first time in my life, I really wanted to give up. It sounds ridiculous, but this person I had become. This bodybuilder. This had become my identity. My reality. I felt like a loser. I think that Mandy was relieved. Perhaps she felt that now I could move on with my life, that we could be more normal without everything revolving around food, training, and bodybuilding drugs. This was the beginning of my downward spiral. I was angry, hurt, and lost and had no idea who I was. I felt like I had blown it, despite trying my hardest. I had started a new adventure. I was on my own personal highway to hell.

CHAPTER 27

Striving for Normality

Normal. I decided I was going to be normal. Mandy and I were out with another couple for dinner. My sometime training partner Mike and his wife, Robin. I remember thinking, "This isn't so bad. Being normal. Out for a nice dinner with friends." Of course, I was placating myself.

We definitely talked about the bodybuilding world, though. Mike and I both agreed that bodybuilding was going in the wrong direction—too much drug use and emphasis on dinosaur-like size. I had already stopped using all steroids and was still training but wasn't training for any reason other than liking being big and strong.

I had started a new job running the training department of a large gym chain. Shortly after that, Mandy and I started house shopping. I was making more money now, and we had slowly paid off most of our debts. We started planning the wedding as well. I suppose all of this was a distraction for me. The result, though, was that Mandy and I never got along better. She liked me just working out for fun. I wasn't so serious all of the time.

Other than spending way too many hours at my new job, our life was good. We found a beautiful house in a nice area in Winnipeg and even got a dog, a yellow lab we named Bella. Not long after, we decided she needed a buddy and got her a pal from the Humane Society, a lab mix I named Rocco, after Rocky Balboa.

On paper, everything was great. Deep inside, my personal demons were still there. They were quiet for the time being.

I really wasn't planning on competing again. However, I was still under contract with Muscletech, and getting all the protein powder I could use for free was still very nice. They wanted me to return to Nationals. Someone there saw some sort of potential in me, even though I could no longer see it. The biggest mistake I had made was going into a show with expectations, which is really foolish in bodybuilding. In my first Nationals, I had zero expectations, so my fourth place finish was a huge personal victory.

The next year, I ASSUMED I would place higher. It is a JUDGED event, so assuming the judges will see it your way is ludicrous, especially when you have no idea who may show up and how good they could look. The judges, after all, select the winner based on their opinion of who looks the best. Unlike the black and white world of Powerlifting. Either you lift the weight, or you don't.

It took many years to wrap my brain around this philosophy. As far as competing that year, I decided to do it. My reasons, however, were much different than before. I pretty much saw it as a paid mini-vacation for Mandy and me. I had never been to Montreal, and being of French heritage, I was excited at the prospect of going there. Mandy was all for it. By all accounts, Montreal had a reputation of being like a European city. We felt it was a win/win. I was honouring my contractual obligations by competing, and we got to have an early honeymoon!

It wasn't that I didn't train for the show. I did. This time around, my approach was very different. There were NO expectations on my part. The other decision I made was to stop using all anabolic steroids. No diuretics or cutting drugs either. Just food and protein powder and training. This is rarely attempted at a National Level show. My goal was simply not to embarrass myself.

As it turns out, I did not embarrass myself at all. The body that I brought to that show was respectable. I was down a little in size as I did not have the steroids to stop my body from losing muscle as I dieted. I also was not as ripped as the previous year. However, I did not look out of place on stage going against National level guys that were juiced to the gills. In the end, I finished 11th, only one spot down from the previous year. As soon as I walked off-stage, I grabbed my cell and messaged Mandy to meet me out front. I didn't stay to see who won or find out my placing (I found out later). I simply did not care. It was freeing to a degree. We spent the next couple of days eating absolutely amazing food and shopping. We had fun.

There would be more changes. I was offered a job as a sales rep for a heating and air conditioning company. It was a lot fewer hours than I was spending at the gym and, in some ways, a lot less draining mentally. I had grown tired of people that wanted to change their bodies but were unwilling to do the work or eat properly so that they could actually achieve their goals. As a person that had spent my life pushing myself physically, I could not relate. Often, the harder the challenge, the better I liked it. If there had been studies to prove that eating dogshit would build muscle and made you look like Arnold, then I would have been choking down dogshit six times a day. These people were whining about not being able to eat bread. Or I would hear things like, "I'm not giving up bacon!" Better yet, they would ask me what was the best booze to drink while trying to lose body fat. They never liked my answer, "water." It felt like a complete waste of time. It was easy to walk away.

Mandy and I got married in a nice little ceremony on a beach in Mexico. It was very small, with only a few people in attendance. We all had a great time. The first warning signs started to pop into my head during the ceremony.

As we were exchanging vows, there was a prominent thought that kept going through my mind, "Wow, I'm really doing this again?"

It did not feel like what I had imagined. I'm an emotional guy. I felt nothing.

The demons were stirring and starting to talk. "What are you doing, man? Is this what you want? You want to be married and sell furnaces and air conditioners? Has been. Worse yet, you are not even that. You are a never was. You will be known as that guy that had potential and did nothing with it."

I ignored my demons for the time being and tried to be normal and happy.

I never understood why sales had to be a complicated song and dance full of bullshit and false promises. Even though my new job was paying me more money than I had ever thought I would make in my life, I was beginning to have some real ethical issues with what I was doing. My job was simple enough in theory. Go into people's homes and assess if they needed either a new furnace or air conditioner or both.

The whole setup started with a lie and went south from there. When people would call our company to set up an appointment, our receptionist was already following a script and the first lie was that the appointment would take about "30 minutes." The truth of the matter was that if the sales rep did everything they were supposed to, following the lengthy script and presentation, the whole thing took two hours minimum. It was horrible.

Their sales process was one that was supposed to build so much fear in the client that everyone did shoddy work (except us, of course) that could possibly endanger the safety of their family and household. It was not a soft sell. You had to beat the customers down until they capitulated.

I think I followed the whole sales process ONCE! After that, I just decided there was no way. I was not going to lie to people. I decided I was going to come in, tell them HONESTLY if they needed new equipment, then explain the costs and go from there. Essentially, treat them as I would like to be treated. If a sales rep came into my house and started going through an elaborate bullshit sales presentation when I simply wanted to know if I needed a new system and the cost, well, I would have tossed him out on his ass. I quickly became one of their top salespeople, following my OWN method of just being honest.

However, the managers would conduct bogus "ride-alongs" on a regular basis. It was their way of making sure you were following the "system." I had a huge problem with this. I did not like being babysat. Often in sales, just like in sports, the manager position is often one with a very high turnover rate. So, every time we got a new manager, and they insisted on coming with me on a ride-along, I would do my best to explain to them that I did things my way and I wasn't going to change. I would definitely use my physical presence to emphasize my point, and very few managers challenged me on it. After all, I was selling, and wasn't that the point?

I knew my days were numbered. It was soul-killing work. There was still a lot of bullshit involved. I remember that during a slow period our manager came up with a brilliant idea to send us door to door, to try and sell furnaces. I looked my manager right in the eye and said, "There is no way I am doing that."

When he could see I was serious, he decided to "let" me just cold call people instead. He wanted me to sit on the phone and try and drum up business. I said sure and proceeded to make zero phone calls. The inner demons got louder. I was unhappy. I could not do normal.

Already Mandy and I were drifting apart and not sleeping in the same bed anymore as she couldn't handle my snoring and nightmares. Instead, I slept with the dogs. I missed having a goal. Money wasn't making me happy. The more I made, the more debt we had. I started to long for competition. Mandy had stopped coming to the gym. I felt she did not understand me. She was spending more time with her friends on the weekends, drinking. She knew how I felt about alcohol, and we definitely had some huge fights over it. I could not stand being around drunks, so I did not handle it well if she got drunk. She was not an alcoholic, but she did drink on a regular basis, as many people do. Unfortunately for me, that was the quickest way to make me fearful and anxious. I hated booze. I hated how people acted because of it and hated that it had robbed me of my father and childhood. Mandy simply expected me to "get over it already."

I withdrew to my safe place—the gym. I started training harder again, watching my food intake.

People started asking questions, "You doing a show, Todd?"

I would always say no and just kept on training.

Another thing was starting to happen. Something I am not proud of, but I started to notice other women. Mandy and I were not as close, and I started to think about what things would be like if I was with a woman that shared my lifestyle.

Another realization popped into my head, my contract with Muscletech was going to expire after Nationals of that year. Along with it, any opportunity to make an extra $2000.00/month for winning a pro card.

I was now 40 years old, which qualified me as a Master. Although the Masters division was a very tough division, if you won it, that qualified you as a pro. The wheels had started to turn. I started a cycle of steroids and began training in earnest. At this point, I kept it to myself. This would not be an easy conversation to have with the wife. I decided to play up the financial aspect of it. I also lied and said that the Masters division was much easier, just a "bunch of old guys."

After a long talk, I sold her on the idea. My inner demons were happy for the time being. This was not going to be like Montreal. I was going all out, pushing my body hard and taking fewer sales calls at work. My focus became competing again. We were trying to make our marriage work, but I think we both knew that we were heading in different directions. I loved Mandy, and I believe she loved me. However, my head was not right. There was still something deep down that was making me crazy. I could not do normal. I had to do this. No matter the cost. I needed to win.

CHAPTER 28

The King and I

It's easy to analyze things in hindsight.

I had to be about 7 or 8 years old. I was in bed asleep when the sound of music woke me from my slumber. Rubbing the sleep out of my eyes, I crept towards the living room. The lights were out, and my Mom was lying on the couch. On the TV was a man in the coolest outfit I had ever seen. A white jumpsuit with a high collar and an eagle across the chest and the eagle was made out of jewels. His hair was jet black. He looked like a cool superhero.

My Mom didn't see me. I stood there silent, watching, totally mesmerized. I had never seen anyone as slick as this guy. Finally, I couldn't help myself, and I very quietly asked my Mom, "Who is that?"

Her answer was spoken so softly, with reverence, "It's Elvis."

I do not know if it was because she was so into what she was watching, but she did not scold me and send me to bed. I quietly snuck onto the living room rocking chair and sat watching just as blown away as she was. The way the people reacted to his every move. His voice was not like anything I had ever heard in my life. I had never seen my Mom impressed by ANYONE before and her eyes never left the TV.

Right then and there, I knew I wanted that. I was used to feeling alone and ignored. I wanted people to react to me the way they reacted to HIM! Mom let me watch the whole concert. In fact, from then on, whenever an Elvis movie was on, she would let me know, and she would let me watch it, even if it was the late movie (which it usually was).

We bonded over Elvis. My Mom loved him, and I did as well. I would wish that he could be my Dad. I would stand on our front steps and belt out Elvis songs to the passing traffic (we lived on a busy street) during rush hour. I would pace the top of our steps like it was my stage. People would smile, and some would applaud if the cars had stopped as they waited for the traffic light to turn green. Elvis was different, and of course, that made me want to be like him.

Our downstairs neighbor was the first to tell us. She knocked on our door, and when my Mom answered, she had tears in her eyes, "Elvis died" was all she could manage, and she burst into tears. My Mom cried as well.

I ran out of the house and jumped on my bike, and rode around and around my block for hours, "NOOOO NOT AGAIN!", these words kept racing through my young mind. "You took my Dad. Now you take my hero?!?" I was mad at God. I hated Him at that moment. I kept riding and crying and singing the words to "You Saw Me Crying in The Chapel" over and over.

It was getting dark, and I had to go home. My Mom was in her room, crying and listening to the radio. Every station was playing only Elvis songs. I asked if I could come in. She nodded. Lying on the foot of the bed, we both cried, listening to our hero sing. It may sound silly, but Elvis brought us both a tremendous amount of joy, and really, we did not have many sources of that in our lives. It was a huge loss at the time. It is a bond that we share to this day, our love of Elvis.

Many years later, now I was on stage, not in a jumpsuit, quite the opposite, almost naked actually. People were calling MY name, cheering for me. Camera flashes were going off. No, it wasn't 50,000 people in attendance, but it may as well have been. It felt like it. I remember thinking, I wish my Mom could see this.

So maybe it was that Elvis concert all those years ago. It was the trigger.

After my Dad's death, I felt very different and odd. I took solace in the fact that Elvis was an outsider when he was in school. He looked different, had wild hair, and was bullied. Well, he had the last laugh, didn't he? Or did he? His success ultimately destroyed him.

I would never experience the adulation that Elvis did. Few in history ever have. We had a couple of things in common, however. We both were strong communicators yet could both be painfully shy. We both experienced bullying and feeling like the odd one out. Last but not least, we could self-destruct like nobody's business especially if we were bored and did not feel challenged.

I was about to travel down a path of self-destruction like I was on a mission. I would destroy everything I loved and kill every relationship that mattered to me. I could not handle success. I was lost. I was mad at God and everything else. As far as I was concerned, I was going to hell faster than a speeding bullet. I figured, "If I'm going, I am going while singing Burning Love!" I wanted to tell everyone to fuck off and get out of the way! Here I am. It's just me, well…and Elvis, the King, and I!

I was losing it.

CHAPTER 29

Careful What You Wish For

It's funny how most of us measure success: a good job, money, a big house, maybe a fancy car. Some envision success of a different sort. Climbing Everest, an Olympic Gold Medal, or perhaps it's fame that we seek. Still, others have to hit rock bottom before achieving any level of success.

I believe some people are set on self-destruct. Sometimes it can be due to the environment in which they developed. Or maybe, that's just the way that some of us are hard-wired. At the time, you could have asked me to give an example of what success looked like, and I could have spouted out a very believable and honourable example of what success in life should look like: Health, family, being happy in one's own skin, a relationship with God and blah blah blah. I could talk. That was my gift. The truth was I had no idea what real success was—no clue as to why I was driven the way I was. Had I reached all my goals, I am quite certain that not only would I have not been able to handle it, but I would also have sabotaged it and found a way to begin the nosedive to my own personal hell anyway!

On the surface, it looked like I was doing well. I had become a master at portraying a caricature of myself. When I wanted to, I could get along with anyone and look as though I had all my shit together. I certainly had all the trappings. Was I rich? Hell no. However, I had a gorgeous wife, a great stepson, a big house, two great dogs, we both drove new cars, and my body looked like something you saw in a comic book. People knew I had an endorsement deal and that I had ONCE competed well at Nationals. I told myself that I had dealt with everything: my past and my anger. Pushing your feelings down and burying them is NOT dealing with them. It's avoidance. Just because you don't see smoke and lava pouring out of a volcano does not mean there is not a shitstorm brewing deep within.

I pushed myself in the gym and took my diet seriously. My anabolic use was at an all-time high. Low compared to many, but I was pushing the envelope, and I knew it. I became determined to do well at Nationals. I added muscle. Rob was also going to compete this year after placing second in the Masters Class, and he was taking things seriously this year. We communicated throughout our prep, encouraging one another.

I was pushing everything else in life to the side: Mandy, Kyle, my job, even my health. I began having severe sleep issues. I would stop breathing several times each night. On top of that, sometimes, I would wake up choking. My throat would close, and I would be fighting for air. The sound it would make was sickening. Mandy and I came up with a system if I woke up choking. I would always run to the bathroom and try to breathe. It was loud, and it always woke her up. She would follow me to the bathroom and ask me over and over if I needed her to call 911. I told her if I ever nod that she was to call immediately.

I would always fight, and to this point, it hasn't killed me. It was insanity. A normal person would go to the doctor. Again, I wasn't normal and definitely wasn't thinking rationally. It would be years before I decided to get checked out by a doctor for this issue. I was afraid the doctor would tell me it was steroid-related, and I did not want to hear that at all. It's not that I wanted to die, but at the same time, I was not going to back off of the gas pedal.

On another occasion, I found myself in the Emergency room due to a bad muscle strain. The doctor asked me what all Doctors ask me, "You take steroids?" I was always open about that with them, no point in lying. I suppose I wasn't looking very healthy because he decided to do some blood work.

When he got the results, he came back into the exam room and asked me a question that I did not expect. "Are you allergic to latex?"

Looking at him confused, I answered, "Um, no. Why?"

He got right to the point, "I would like you to call your wife. You have pancreatitis. If we do not get this under control, you are going to be in trouble, so we have to be prepared for the possibility of emergency surgery. It is most likely caused by your steroid use."

You would think that hearing that would have made me rethink the choices I was making. In reality, what I was thinking was, "This is not going to be a fun phone call to Mandy." Luckily, they were able to stabilize everything, and they let me go home the next day.

Mandy was not happy. She was worried. Understandably so.

I told her I would back off the steroids. I did cut back. Probably not enough, and the choking and sleep apnea continued. I had blinders on. She was trying, God bless her, but I could not or would not hear her. My demons were in control now.

I think it's common for bodybuilders to think, "Nobody understands what we go through!" There is a lot of truth to that. To be honest, what we do to ourselves is, for lack of a better term, crazy. We take drugs in amounts that can potentially harm us in an effort to look "uber-healthy." See the irony?

Nationals were being held in Toronto that year, and I was excited at the prospect of competing there. It felt more like the "big time" as opposed to competing in Winnipeg. Montreal had that same feel, but because I really did not try to be competitive for that show, it really did feel more like a vacation than a contest. This felt intense and important.

We hit a small snag leading up to the show. We could not find anyone to watch the dogs while we would be away. At least that's how I remember it. In hindsight, I don't think Mandy wanted to go. The whole year had stressed her terribly, with my focus being on anything but our life together. Perhaps she had enough of it all. My tunnel vision was so bad that it really did not bother me that she wasn't going.

"One less thing for me to worry about" was my thinking at the time. Bodybuilding is a very selfish endeavour, after all.

When I arrived at the host hotel, I texted Rob right away to see if he was there yet. He was and gave me his room number. It would be good to see my friend, and I was thrilled that we would both be competing in our respective best conditions. When I got to his room, I was completely shocked by what I saw when he opened the door. He was completely covered up, EXCEPT his forearms. His forearms were so lean it looked like someone had pulled his skin off. His face was completely devoid of any and all fat and was completely sunk in.

I had seen Rob ripped before, but this was a new inhuman level I did not think was possible. Any thoughts I had of beating him (if he won the light class of the masters and I won the heavy class, we would have had to battle it out for the overall title) quickly vanished.

"Holy crap, Rob!" was all I could manage.

He laughed and then asked if I wanted to see what the rest of him looked like.

I really did not, because his forearms alone destroyed me. As his friend, I knew he would like my honest opinion, so he stripped down to his trunks and hit a few poses. At that point in my competitive career, I had never been as blown away by someone's condition as I was at that moment.

He asked me if I had seen Sandy Rideout yet, who Rob felt could be a possible threat. Sandy was also known for freaky conditioning. I had, in fact, bumped into Sandy earlier, and he looked great. Rob, on the other hand, looked like an alien life form.

"I seen Sandy, he looks great, but you're going to destroy him."

Rob seemed relieved to hear that.

Then he asked me, "Ok, let's see how you look."

I was reluctant. I was in shape for sure, but nothing like him.

He kept on, "C'mon, I can tell by your face. You are ready."

I stripped down and hit a few shots.

He nodded approvingly, "You are going to do really well. You look great!"

It was good to hear it, of course, because I knew he was giving an honest opinion, but I still realized that as good as I was, there was another level, and I was not there yet.

At the weigh-in, I saw the fellows I would be going up against. I gulped hard. Everyone looked great. Every last one of them. This class was no cakewalk. It was filled with very seasoned guys that all had been very close to turning pro.

Leon "The Beast" Eastman was in my class along with Tyrone Ashmeade, two very large guys that definitely had come to win. Another monster was Ludvik Rolin, who had out-weighed me by at least 25 lbs. He was huge. I composed myself as a photographer gathered the whole class for a group picture.

"To hell with it, I thought. These guys don't scare me. I'm in shape. I am going to do well!"

It was odd being there by myself. In the hotel room, I called Mandy. She seemed distant when we spoke. I was losing her. At the time, it was like my emotions had withered away. It didn't bother me other than harbouring some resentment that she had not made the trip. There WAS a part of me that still cared, my last bit of humanity.

After the phone call, I took not one but two different diuretics. One of which, Lasix, was known to be quite dangerous if used improperly. The side effects, severe cramping, and if you took too much, well, you could die. I was determined to shed my body of every last drop of water that might obscure my muscular definition.

I would spend the night urinating every 20 minutes. Along with the other drug, it proved to be too much for my system. The next morning, I woke up and stretched, flexing my legs as I did so. The pain was intense and immediate! Both legs completely seized up along with my abdominal muscles. I screamed from the shock, or rather, yelped. I was frozen. I could not move at all. I had brought a bottle of potassium pills just in case I had a problem with cramping, but it was on the nightstand out of my reach.

My heart was racing in my chest. I quickly realized that I was in big trouble. People died from this shit. I did not wish to become bodybuilding's next casualty. With every bit of strength that I could muster, I tried to push my abdominal muscles back into place. That didn't work. So, inch by inch, I worked my way closer and closer to the nightstand and the potassium pills. Finally, I got close enough to grab the bottle and quickly swallowed a couple of pills and tried to relax. Slowly, my heart rate returned to normal, and the muscles unfroze. It took me 15 minutes to work my way to those pills and several more minutes until I could stand up. When I could, I went to the full-length mirror and took a look to see how my condition was. I smiled at my reflection. The Lasix almost killed me, but damn if it didn't work! I was careful not to flex too much as I did not want to risk cramping up a second time.

It was time to carb up with a good breakfast before the show. I made my way to the hotel restaurant that overlooked a beautiful hotel swimming pool. I ordered pancakes and bacon and eggs. I was there early, and no other bodybuilders had yet come down for breakfast.

The chef came over and introduced himself as Romel. He himself was a successful bodybuilder, and we had a great conversation about contest prepping and how hard the diet could be. I had confessed that more than anything, I missed cookies and milk. We had a good laugh. It often was the simplest foods that one misses, and we both agreed on that point. He made me a fantastic breakfast and told me to come back after the show and that he would make something up special for me!

Finally, it was time to head over to the venue. Rob, his wife Asha, and their baby girl and I all headed over together. Rob was in great spirits, as he should be. He knew he was going to win. You could see it on his face.

Rob's class was up first. He won easily. Now it was our turn to see who Rob would have to face for the overall Masters Title. I strode onto the stage with confidence. My body was much bigger and a whole lot leaner than it was in Montreal. This was no vacation. The judges ran us through our poses, and I was hitting them with confidence when all of a sudden, my left calf completely seized up with a cramp. It hurt like hell. I slowly stretched it out in between poses and gave zero indication that I was having an issue. I kept posing and smiling, all the while praying to the Bodybuilding Gods that be, that I didn't completely seize up on stage. I got through the prejudging, and it was very evident that I was in the top three with Tyrone Ashmeade and Leon "The Beast."

Later that evening, when they called out the top three finalists, I was happy to see that I was not mistaken and was in that group. I finished third, Tyrone second, and Leon first. Rob went on to beat Leon for the overall win and his pro card. I was so happy for him and glad that we went through the journey together.

I couldn't help but think, "Next year, I am winning this thing!" For now, though, I was happy. I had proven to myself once again that I could hang with the big boys and beat guys that were much bigger than myself.

As soon as I got to my hotel room, I called Mandy. I was excited to tell her how I did. When she answered the phone, I could hear a lot of background noise, she had friends over, and they were deep into the wine.

"Babe, I got THIRD!"

She answered back, "What?" people were talking to her, and she seemed distracted.

I told her again, and she replied with a "Way to go!" and then explained that her friends were over and we would talk more tomorrow.

It hurt. I had wanted her to be proud of me. Excited as I was, I got what I deserved. I had really pulled away from her during that year, and truthfully, I had no right to be hurt. She was doing her own thing. So, there I was, alone with my trophy. I ordered some pizza and watched some TV. The happiness had left. Even my demons were quiet.

My flight did not leave until Monday, so that meant I had a full day to myself in Toronto. Almost all of the competitors had started to leave on Sunday, so it was nice and quiet. I went back to the restaurant and had a nice breakfast, then decided that I would get my bathing suit on and hang by the gorgeous pool. It was really a great setup. From the pool area, you had a fantastic view of the harbour as well as the CN Tower.

After a few minutes one of the most beautiful women that I had ever seen walked up to me and started a conversation. She had competed the day before and was at the pool for a photoshoot. She was charming and absolutely stunning to look at. When her photographer showed up, she excused herself, but before she did, she gave me her contact info and told me that I should "get in touch."

I lay down on my lounger and watched as this beautiful young woman went through various poses during her photoshoot. It was sunny and warm. I had just placed third the day before, and I remember thinking, "This is a perfect moment. It can't get better than this!" And then, it did!

"Excuse me, sir?"

I looked up to see a young waiter holding a tray with a plate full of chocolate chip cookies and a large glass of milk.

"Compliments of Chef Romel, he baked these for you."

So, there I sat, eating fresh baked cookies, drinking milk while watching a Goddess pose in the sun. It was an absolute pure moment of joy.

A thought crossed my mind, "Maybe I SHOULD get a girl like that." I think deep down inside, my demons were laughing. This moment was to be, in many ways, the high point of my bodybuilding career. There is an old saying, "Be careful what you wish for." But for right now, at this moment, for one day, I had found peace. It would be a long time before I would experience peace again.

CHAPTER 30

Nowhere to go but...

I was pretty damn pleased with myself after pacing 3rd at the Canadian Bodybuilding Championships. My success had completely squashed the fear that had started to plague me, namely, that my fourth place finish in 2006 was a fluke. Finishing top 3 was an indication to me that not only could I hang at that level, I could win.

My sights were now firmly set on just that, training another year all out with the goal of winning Nationals and turning pro in 2010. Everything had started to shift. My reasons for training in the first place, my personal belief system, what was important to me. Artistry? What's that? Family? Career? It all started to slip away.

There are many that say that anabolic use does not really affect a person's mental state or outlook. That it only affects the physical. Yes, in some individuals, there can be increased levels of aggressive behaviour. I, of course, refer them to the "asshole rule." If you're an asshole, to begin with, you will just be a bigger (literally and figuratively) asshole on the juice. Steroids affected me differently. As I increased my dosage, I did not get angry or impatient. Instead, I grew cold. I cared less. Much less. Going through the motions is perhaps the best way to describe it. I was only feeling alive when in the gym.

When I arrived home from Toronto, I could sense that things were changing at home. While I was overjoyed with my performance, Mandy did not really seem to care. That did not sadden me. It was more like, "She doesn't get it. How could she understand?"

What I was feeling was more like resentment and anger towards her, to be truthful. She had done nothing wrong. If I had to guess, looking back, she had probably just had enough. Instead of talking to her about it, I removed myself emotionally from the situation. She started spending more time with her friends drinking wine as I stayed home and stewed about it. It was her fault she didn't get it. At least, that is what I told myself.

Things really ended for Mandy and me on a cold night in January. Mandy was at her friend's house drinking until the wee hours. I was getting worried. Alcohol still made me uneasy, and whenever she would be out drinking late, it put me into a bad mental space. Perhaps it sounds cliché, but after what I experienced as a child, I would never feel comfortable around situations that involved booze. I took it personally that even though Mandy knew my fears and concerns regarding the subject, she pretty much just ignored it and did what she wanted to anyway.

There had been many fights about it over the course of our relationship. In fact, we almost ended before we got serious when she got very drunk at my work Christmas party, and I had to drag her out of there before she made a spectacle of herself. Like many people, if Mandy had too much to drink, her logic and common sense went right out the window along with any filter as to what she said. It bothered me to no end that at this stage of my life, I had to worry about my wife drinking too much.

On this particular night, I received a panicked text at 3:00 am from her friend explaining that "Mandy was drunk and had left her house to walk home." I completely lost my shit on her friend. It was 3:00 am. She's drunk, wearing heels, walking in the snow, and it -30 degrees outside.

"WHY THE FUCK DIDN'T YOU STOP HER!" I screamed.

"You know how she gets," was her only reply.

I got into my car and raced off in the direction of her friend's house.

Thoughts of terrible outcomes were racing through my mind. One of the kids I went to high school with had died doing the same thing. I still remembered his name, Steven Dee. He had gotten drunk at a party and passed out on the way home and froze to death. I tried to shake such images out of my rage-filled mind.

A few minutes later, I saw her, stumbling down the road, very drunk. I flagged her down, and she got into the car, kind of laughing. I wasn't laughing. I was shaking with rage. The fight didn't happen until the next day when she was sober. It was awful. We screamed at each other, both of us quite sure that the other was wrong.

It was not long after that incident that we decided to split up. That was it. One year of marriage after almost six years of being together. I didn't care. I wanted my bodybuilding life. As much as I hate to admit this, I had started talking and flirting with a female competitor from the gym.

"She would understand me," was my thinking at the time, "she lives the same lifestyle as me."

It was, of course, a band-aid. I started seeing Denise before I had even moved out. Mandy and I were being amicable. I justified it in my mind by telling myself, "It's ok, you and Mandy are done, you can move on."

I did not want Mandy to find out, but of course, she did, and all hell broke loose. Mandy was and is a great young lady. She raised an amazing young man in Kyle. She did not deserve any of this. Truthfully, it did not even have anything to do with her. I had never dealt with all my garbage. I just pushed it down. Now it was exploding in all of its destructive splendour. I could justify everything. It wasn't my fault after all.

My world was blowing up, and everyone could see it except me. I walked away from a wonderful wife and stepson, a nice home, her family, and everything we had built together. I felt almost nothing. I would train and win Nationals. I would be somebody. I wasn't normal after all, right? My demons laughed. Blind. I was blind. I could not see that I WAS somebody.

I had been sucked into a hole of selfishness and wasn't even training for the right reasons anymore. Gone was the art form, replaced by my need for a trophy, a pro card, and recognition—my need to prove something to the world. But it wasn't the world really; it was to me. It was simply too hard for me to believe I was anything good. Mandy loved me, and I could not deal with it even though it was, in fact, the one thing I wanted the most.

I remember standing in our living room for the very last time after I had packed the last of my things. It really was a beautiful home, on a quiet street, in a very nice neighborhood. As a child, I had dreamt of living in a home like this.

"This is the last time I will see this place," I thought to myself. I let out a deep sigh. There was not a lot of my humanity left by this point. Just enough, though, to make me feel something. For a brief second, I allowed myself to acknowledge what I was losing and the pain I had caused Mandy and Kyle. I could not allow that emotion to grab hold of me, and I pushed it down. Just like I always did.

"Shoulder down?" I thought, but it wasn't the same. I don't think Coach K would have approved of anything I had been doing.

"Nowhere to go but…." my thought trailed off. The inner demons were winning. I think they were trying to destroy me.

"Nahhhh, I got this." And with that, I walked out of our home and proceeded to begin my journey to full-blown self-destruction!

CHAPTER 31

"If I can walk out of here, I'm competing!"

I decided the best way to move forward was to not look back at all. I dove into a relationship with Denise right away, and in some ways, I had been right. It was easier to live with someone that lived the same bodybuilding lifestyle. We had one thing in common, our lifestyle. We ate the same, trained together, and had similar goals.

We had moved in together, renting a small house in the community of St. Norbert. I still had Rocco, but Mandy and I had found a new home for Bella as I did not know where I was going to end up and wasn't sure if I could have even one dog, let alone two. Rocco was sad without Bella, so Denise and I adopted a 10-week-old puppy from a rescue. He turned out to be a Rottweiler cross and was not only a great dog but he and Rocco became the best of pals. I named him Apollo, after Apollo Creed from the movie "ROCKY."

Our life was simple. Have sex, eat, train, and repeat. Denise was a lot younger than me, and other than training, eating, and sex, we really had nothing in common. That being said, she was very good to me, as were her parents. We even went out to their cabin a few times and often had family dinners together. For the time being, this was enough. The demons had once again been silenced. They were probably just patiently waiting to see what the next step in my path of self-destruction would be.

It really didn't take long. I still had my sales rep job but had further decreased the number of sales calls I took so that I could focus more on training. It was during one of my sales calls that I met Aubrey. Even though Denise was very good to me, I had still shut off the capacity to truly love. I was ignoring the pain I was in. Everything that was killing me inside was still being pushed aside. No matter how well Denise treated me, I was not happy or satisfied. Some people use booze or drugs to mask pain. I was using female attention.

I liked Aubrey right away. She was physically beautiful and physically strong as well. She trained and wanted to compete. I could not stop myself from flirting with her, and even after the sales call was over, we stayed in touch. We started making plans to get together. Finally, we had an opportunity. Denise was going to a bridal shower, so I made plans with Aubrey. She invited me over.

However, when I arrived at her house, she wasn't there. I texted her only to find out she had made alternate plans and we would have to try for another time. I was not impressed, but what could I do? For a brief moment, I thought, "Man, maybe this is a sign. You know it's not right. You have no reason to cheat on Denise. She's an awesome girlfriend. Maybe God is trying to tell you something, and this might be a second chance to do the right thing." I quickly pushed those thoughts aside and began the 25-minute drive home.

The van tore through my car with such ferocity I was completely stunned for several seconds before I realized what had happened. A large cargo van had run a red light and completely tore through the front end of my car. Every airbag had gone off as my car was thrown into another vehicle after the initial impact. Once I had regained my senses, I became aware of an intense pain in my head and neck as well as my left shoulder.

The interior of my car had started to fill with smoke, and I thought, "Oh hell no!"

I tried to open the door to no avail. It wouldn't budge—more smoke. I tried the other door. No good. Panic started to set in. Then anger.

"Nope! Not today! I am NOT going out like this!!!" I braced myself, then opened the door handle, and as hard as I could, rammed my injured left shoulder into the driver's side door. It popped open. I half fell out of the car and stood up. I took a few steps forward and then looked back at my completely crushed front end. I loved that car. It was a black fully loaded Honda Accord V6 coupe.

The next emotion I felt was rage. I turned around and started looking for the vehicle that hit me. There it was, a large white cargo van. I started walking toward it, my head filled with thoughts of retribution and payback. I remember thinking, "I am going to completely dismantle the motherfucker that did this!"

My blind rage was quickly replaced by blackness. I woke up seated in someone's sport utility vehicle. Some kind-hearted people had stopped and picked me up off the ground, and apparently, I half walked into their vehicle, where they tried to keep me awake until the ambulance arrived.

The next thing I remember was being strapped to a board and the ride in the ambulance. I managed to text Denise. During the ride to the hospital, the emergency responders tried to keep me awake, asking me questions like, "So, you're a bodybuilder, hey?"

I answered, mumbling, "Yeah, I am competing at the Canadian Championships in a week and a half."

I vaguely remember the EMT replying, "Um, let's just make sure you're okay, buddy."

Once at the hospital, I was brought into an examining room and given the once over. I was wheeled into the X-ray department and then afterward a CAT scan. After the tests, I was wheeled back into an examining room. I once again tried texting Denise, but I think she was under the impression that I was just in a fender bender. I was alone for a moment and felt the urge to urinate, so I got up and began filling the bottle they provided for that very thing.

Just as I finished, a nurse came in and shouted at me, "What are you doing? Do NOT get up! Do not move! You have a head and neck injury!"

I decided to text my cousin Sherry. She was the only relative from my Dad's side that I had communication with. We had reconnected in recent years, and strangely enough, she had competed in physique contests as well. She came to the hospital right away, and it was comforting having her there.

Shortly after she arrived, the Doctor came in and gave me very clear instructions, "Todd, we are going to remove your neck brace, then we are going to place this heavier duty one on you. Now, it is VERY important that you do not move. Do not try and help us. Just let us fit the new brace on you." He spoke slowly and carefully.

I looked up at Sherry. Her look was one of concern. I was in a lot of pain, but up until that point, I really was not worried. I was wondering, "What is going on?"

Once they had the new brace on, the Doctor continued, "Todd, listen carefully. According to the X-rays, it looks like your neck is broken, so it is very important that you do not move at all until we tell you it's okay to do so. Do you understand?"

Hearing those words was very much like being punched in the stomach. I felt a tear run down the side of my face as I assured the Doctor I would not move. Sherry was doing her best to comfort me, but I could hear the panic in her voice. All of a sudden, the thought of competing in bodybuilding did not seem like such a big deal. It was completely minimized by the thought of spending the rest of my life as a cripple. I was wheeled away for more scans and tests.

After what seemed like an eternity, the Doctor came back. "Good news, your neck is not broken, there is an abnormality in your spine, and you have a concussion, but you will be okay. We will keep you here tonight to monitor you."

A wave of relief washed over me. As the Doctor started to walk away, I called out to him, "Does this mean I can still compete in a week and a half?"

He looked at me like I was insane. "Compete? I don't think so. You've taken a pretty good beating tonight. I highly doubt you will even be able to move properly for at least a couple of weeks."

As I laid there, I started to get angry. "No way. I have gone through too much. If I can walk out of here, I'm competing! This is nothing!" Against Doctor's orders, I was back in the gym two days later.

CHAPTER 32

"I'm just tired."

The funny thing about a blow to the head is that quite simply, you never know how it's going to affect you. Perhaps returning to the gym immediately after my car accident was not the wisest decision in the world. However, many athletes will simply soldier on through adversity, even if it means possible self-harm. It's the way we are wired. We are conditioned to ignore the pain and simply push through it. Take the NFL, for example. We are now seeing many retired NFL players dealing with dementia, not to mention a host of other physical ailments. The human body can only endure so much after all. Yet, we as athletes do not think of what our quality of life will be like after our athletic careers are finished or the possible long-term ramifications as we are willing, quite literally, to risk our own well-being to win at all costs.

The blackouts started almost immediately after I was released from the hospital. The first one occurred as I was sitting on the couch. Denise thought that I had dozed off. We were talking, and then, just like that, I was out cold. My reaction was to dismiss it. Giving it no more thought other than, "That was weird." That's how it would go. One minute I was talking, the next, I was out cold. I ignored it. "I'm just tired," was what I would keep telling myself. I kept training, sticking to my diet as Nationals was fast approaching.

I finally acknowledged there might be a problem when I woke up as the rental car that I was driving bounced off the centre median. There was no warning. I decided that once I got back from competing, I would get checked out by a Doctor. That would have to wait as I did not want to hear from anyone that competing was a bad idea. One of the scarier things that would sometimes occur after these episodes would be paralysis. I would black out, wake up from it, and even though I was completely aware of what was going around me, I could not move at all. I could breathe and speak. I could feel. But nothing would work. As in, I literally could not lift a finger. This would last for several minutes and was, in a word, terrifying. Still, I was going to compete come hell or high water. A little thing like blacking out with momentary paralysis was not going to stop me. What an idiot.

Upon arriving at the weigh-in, I was pleased to see many familiar faces. After all, this was now my fifth National event. One begins to make friendships with other athletes, and the officials will start to remember you, especially if you are one of the athletes that finishes well.

As I registered and received my competitor info and number, I was flattered when Helen Bouchard, an IFBB Pro Bodybuilder, said, "Hi Todd, how are you?"

People were starting to know who I was. I ran into MuscleMag writer and photographer Garry Bartlett, and we had a nice little chat about my accident. The previous year he had written about my 3rd place finish and had included a photo with it as well. It was an honour to be in MuscleMag, even if it was just a paragraph and a photo. After hearing about my accident, Garry promised to write about my journey and include it in the issue that covered this show. He was good to his word, and once again, I was thrilled to see my name and photo on the pages of my favourite Bodybuilding magazine.

It was at the athletes' meeting that it happened. Mark Smishek, the President of the CBBF, was addressing the athletes when I passed out cold in my chair. When I snapped out of it, I quickly realized that the paralysis had set in. This only happened about 50% of the time. I sat there terrified.

Out of my peripheral vision, I could see a female competitor that was seated next to me lean towards me. "Are you ok?" she whispered.

"Yeah, I'm just tired," was all I could come up with. I was completely immobile and could feel a trickle of sweat running down the side of my face. I prayed in my head that Mark would keep on talking until I could move again. Finally, after what seemed like an eternity, my mobility returned.

A panicked thought entered my head, "Oh Lord, please do not let me pass out onstage!"

It was going to be a tough show. Both Leon and Tyrone were back, along with a new monster. Chris White from Ontario. He looked amazing. Big, with great shape and conditioning as well. During prejudging, it became apparent that Chris would win with Tyrone and myself battling it out for 2nd and 3rd with Leon right on our heels.

When they called out the top three, it was Tyrone, Chris, and me. I knew I wasn't going to beat Chris, but I felt I had better conditioning and overall balance than Tyrone. He had the edge on me with upper body size, though.

I was holding my breath, hoping to not hear my name called in the third spot: "3rd place…from Manitoba, Todd Payette!"

I waved and bowed to the crowd and judges as I accepted my trophy. It was the toughest show I had been in, and there was no shame in coming in third to these two champions. I made up my mind that I needed to train even harder for the next year's event. Maybe the accident had affected my condition as well. That was what I was telling myself. I would not consciously acknowledge that along with the passing out and the paralysis, I was also having trouble concentrating at times. I was forgetting things and often felt very lost and confused. That all got swept under the proverbial rug under the heading of "I'm just tired, it's just the prep. I am fine."

I was not fine. The cracks in the armour that had been my body were becoming more and more apparent even if I would not acknowledge them.

When I arrived home, I finally decided to make an appointment with a Doctor. Denise was insistent that I do so. To be honest, if not for her, I probably would not have bothered. She wouldn't let it go, and I relented. There was a walk-in clinic within walking distance of our house, so I decided to go there.

After listening to all my symptoms and a brief examination, the Doctor told me that he was sending me to a neurologist for tests. I asked him if he had any idea what could be wrong with me. It was his theory that I was suffering from a type of narcolepsy (which is a type of epilepsy), and it may have been brought on by the car accident.

"That can happen?" I asked.

"Trauma to the head can do many things to the brain," he explained. He also told me that he could revoke my driver's licence as I was now a hazard to the safety of myself and others, should I pass out driving again. In the end, he decided not to if I promised to take a break from driving until we had everything sorted out. He wrote out a note to my employer as I obviously could not work in this condition.

You needed to drive to go to sales calls, and I can imagine that passing out and being paralyzed in front of customers would be frowned upon. I agreed to his terms and went on my way.

Of course, through all of this, I continued to train. Already I was thinking about competing at Nationals in 2011. My world was really slipping away. Nothing else mattered. I don't think I would have stopped even if the Doctor had said there is a 50/50 chance that training and taking steroids will kill you.

I couldn't work, so I decided to train more clients until I could resume work again, as I had been slowly picking up personal training clients over the years. As far as my regular job, well, we had yet another new manager. He had made it clear that he was a "by the book" individual. Which pretty much ensured that we were never going to see eye to eye. When I was into my third week of "recovering" from the car accident, he called me on the phone to fire me. He had no just cause to do this. However, he did it anyway and did so without giving me a solid reason or notice. He didn't like me, and he certainly did not like me being off work and saw it as an excuse to can my ass. He was a weasel, and firing me by phone was just his style, as he really did not have the balls to do it in person. That said, I do not really blame him for letting me go. I was already working on a reduced schedule. My heart wasn't in it, and I certainly had no interest in following the company's policies and guidelines—not to mention their silly ass script! I decided to turn my focus to training people full-time as I could not drive anyway.

Success in bodybuilding can often (but not always) mean that people will hire you to give them the body they always wanted. As I now found myself needing as many clients as possible to support myself, my dogs, as well as the increasing costs associated with bodybuilding at a higher level, I was not overly picky about who I would train. Most of my client base consisted of guys that wanted to get bigger as well as people that wanted to compete in bodybuilding. Many of my clients were already using steroids, which of course, led to the most common thing in the world of bodybuilding—the selling of steroids.

Almost every competitive bodybuilder, at one time or another, will sell steroids. Sometimes it's to their friends, training partners, or people that they train. The bigger and more jacked you are, the more people ask you what you are using as it obviously must be working. The average individual will rarely take into consideration that just maybe, the huge bodybuilder they are buying from has superior genetics, trains harder, and eats better than they do. People really want to believe that the only thing stopping them from being the "next big deal" can be found in a pill or an injection. No matter what you TELL THEM, they do not want to hear it. So, the selling of steroids can be a very easy way for the competitive bodybuilder to cover the costs of their own steroid use as well as help pay for food, cost of living, and everything else that makes being a bodybuilder a money-losing endeavour. Before I knew it, I was getting a fair number of my clients and some of the bodybuilders I knew, their "supps." I wasn't getting rich from the sale of steroids, but it certainly offset the cost of my own.

I was becoming someone else. My whole identity was becoming bodybuilding. I started to see myself as some sort of badass. I grew up respecting the law, wanting to do the right things in life. Now I had become cold and uncaring. Like an animal. A predator.

The things I was doing were not right. I had started seeing Aubrey romantically while still living with Denise. I did have feelings for Aubrey. There was something that drew me to her. Even though I knew what I was doing was wrong, I did it anyway. I did not even try and justify it to myself. I just did it.

I also began to associate with people I would never have associated with before. Through a mutual acquaintance, I was introduced to some very "connected" individuals that wanted training plans and, of course, steroids. They liked how I looked. I trained with them on occasion, and they admired my strength as well. They took me into their inner circle to a degree, and I did not mind. After all, we all wanted to be big and strong. Alpha males. I didn't party with them even though I was invited to many times. The part of me that feared alcohol and rec drugs was still very much a part of who I was.

Even though I was still suffering from blackouts, I decided to blow off my appointment with the neurologist and just proceed with my plans to compete at Nationals. "I'm fine," was the lie that kept me going. I started driving again. I started to notice that there was a warning sign before I passed out—a slight tingling in my head. If I felt it, I had maybe 20 seconds to pull over and just let the blackout occur. I had become pretty good at it. The fear of driving was now a thing of the past.

My life was spiraling out of control at a geometric rate. My time was spent (in no particular order) training, eating, having sex, getting steroids for clients, writing training plans, training clients or one of the boys, and sleeping. I was ignoring all the pain from my life and masking it with everything else. There was a tiny voice in my head that I would hear on occasion that said, "Who are you? You are going to kill yourself, Todd. This isn't you. Do you want to die?"

Sometimes I would answer that voice with, "I don't care."

When a person doesn't care is when that person becomes the most dangerous animal they can be. I no longer cared. I was becoming dangerous to myself and anyone that associated with me. The interesting thing about not giving a shit is that you will do things that are not only outside of your character but, quite possibly, completely idiotic. I had wanted to leave Winnipeg for as long as I could remember, and I started to toss around the idea of moving out West.

Winnipeg is a notoriously frugal city, and I realized that with my background, I could make a lot more money as a trainer in a larger city. Calgary was my first choice. I had decided to take a drive there and investigate the possibility of working out of Golds Gym as a trainer. It was during a conversation I had with one of the "connected guys" I was training that I mentioned I would be away for a day or two as I was headed to Calgary.

"Calgary? Hey, would you mind bringing back a package from there for me? I have a buddy out there, and I don't trust couriers or the mail. I will flip you some bucks for the trouble."

I thought nothing of it, "Yeah, man, all good. Just give your bro my number. As long as I am not driving all over the place, it's cool."

So off I went, driving to Calgary. During the drive, I found myself having to occasionally stop and let a blackout occur. I felt like Spider-Man. When my "Spider-Sense" tingled, I would pull over to avoid passing out while driving. I made it to Calgary safely. I messaged my guy in Winnipeg, and he messaged his friend, and he met me and gave me a package to bring back.

We had a brief conversation about, "How can I get jacked like you." And then I headed to a hotel to crash for the night. The next day I went to Golds to check it out and train. It was a decent enough gym with a good clientele. One of their trainers was a National level competitor that recognized me from Nationals. We chatted, and she introduced me to the manager. We spoke about the possibility of me working there and all in all things were looking good. I checked out of the hotel and headed back to Winnipeg.

"Yeah, Calgary. I think it might be a good fit!" The drive home was uneventful other than my "blackout breaks."

Once home, I discussed the possibility of moving to Calgary with Denise. She was on the fence about it, but I figured over time, she would come around. If she didn't, I didn't really care. Only my selfish goals mattered to me at this point.

I messaged my "buddy" to let him know I was back, and I had his package. We arranged to meet for coffee. We chatted, and I handed him the package, which was a box about the size of a shoebox. He opened it in front of me. It was full of Blackberry cell phones.

"Want one? Give you a great deal on it!" he offered.

I refused as I had just got my first Blackberry not two weeks before.

"Damn, I missed out!" was my thought.

Other than that, I never thought about it again. Funny how life works. I WAS tired. I think many people could see what was coming. Of course, I was oblivious to it all. I was blindly moving forward towards this goal of winning at Nationals. It was my Holy Grail. Like somehow, it would make me whole and give me an identity I could be proud of, make my mother proud. I was dying inside. I had let everything that meant anything slip away. My own self-hatred was destroying me. My demons were winning. I never spoke to God at all. There was no belief in anything. Like a starving man searching for food, I was searching for validation. I had taken something I loved, the beautiful act of training and building your physique, which had been an artistic endeavour to me at one time, and had twisted it into some strange and grotesque fantasy of being the cure-all for a lifetime of pain.

I had strange fantasies of winning at Nationals and then pulling out a small revolver (where the hell I was going to hide it was beyond me) and blowing my brains out right there on stage. "They would never forget that!" was my thought at the time. Maybe the car accident had affected me more than I thought, was I damaged? Or was it a combination of the steroids AND the head trauma? These were questions I would sometimes ask myself in rare moments of lucidity. I would think about getting help and then quickly dismiss those thoughts. I would always replace those thoughts with one simple sentence: "I'm just tired."

CHAPTER 33

"Mr. Swayze, I'm so sorry!"

Before I delve into the deep end of the pool, so to speak, I thought I would share some lighter moments that have occurred in my life simply because, well, I'm a bodybuilder. Let's face it, walking around with arms bigger than many people's legs and low percentages of body fat make an individual stand out in a crowd.

Don't get me wrong, I am not saying being muscular makes a person superior in any way. People, as a rule, respond to anything that is different. Even though weight training is more commonplace than it has ever been in history, a bodybuilder's physique still lands him/her in the vast minority.

Generally, as a rule, most people have the common sense to not say every ignorant or insulting thought that pops into their heads. There are exceptions to that rule, of course. For some reason, society seems to think that making fun of very fit or large muscular bodies is completely acceptable. It's as if they believe that somehow having muscle makes one impervious to insults or ridicule. As if a muscular person has no feelings. Or perhaps they think we are deaf.

I am always amazed at some of the things that have been said while I am clearly within earshot or right to my face. Early on in my career as a "bodybuilder," I decided that I would not tolerate rude behaviour on any level, which has led to some very entertaining situations. Sometimes just being big and strong can lead to funny and sometimes scary situations as well.

Here are just a few instances that may shed some light on what it is like to live life every day as a "bodybuilder!"

"He probably has a small dick!"

Ah yes, my favourite bodybuilding myth. Bodybuilders, or let's say, guys that take steroids, "have small penises." Here is the reality. When you take testosterone or a testosterone-based anabolic steroid, the body will either slow down or stop its own natural production of testosterone. Basically, the body strives for balance. So, if an individual is taking it from an outside source, the body sees no reason to produce it, and it shuts down its production of the hormone. Which, in turn, will cause the TESTICLES to atrophy. The degree to which this happens depends on the individual. It does NOT affect the size of one's penis. SO, if you are small/big without steroids, you will be small/big on steroids. No change. Also, while taking the steroids, one will often have a higher sex drive (as I was to find out). Once off the drugs, as a rule, your own test production will return to normal. In some cases, with prolonged use, you may damage your body's ability to produce sufficient testosterone on its own, which means that you will be taking testosterone replacement for the rest of your life! Still, people love to use this myth as an insult to muscular individuals.

So, without further delay, story number one!

I had walked into a local coffee shop not far from my house. It was a summer day, hot. I was simply picking up an Iced Cappuccino. I happened to be wearing a tank top. When you are muscular, that can be enough to set some people off.

As I was ordering, I could hear a young couple in the corner snickering at me. It was obvious they were laughing at me as I could make out the words "steroids" and "gorilla." It wasn't until I CLEARLY heard the guy say, "He probably has a small dick," that I decided enough was enough.

I told the girl at the till, "Excuse me, I will be right back," and casually walked over to the couple. Then, without saying a word, I positioned myself directly in front of the girl and began undoing my belt and then my pants.

"Dude! What the hell? What are you doing?" the guy said with more than a bit of panic in his voice.

"I'm showing your girlfriend here my dick. You seemed pretty convinced that it must be small, so I figured I would end the debate and pull it out for her."

I then proceeded to reach in my pants as though I was going to pull it out.

"STOP! NO DON'T!" he was now visibly upset. His girlfriend had a very amused look on her face. I zipped up and turned towards him.

I spoke in a deep and serious tone, "Listen, asshole, first things first, I'm big, not deaf. Second, show some respect. How does it feel, being embarrassed like this?"

His cheeks were red with embarrassment.

"Third, I STRONGLY advise you to apologize to me right now!"

At this point, everyone in the coffee shop was watching this little scenario unfold.

"I'm sorry," he quietly muttered.

"I'm sorry, I didn't catch that. Could you speak up? Big guys are often hard of hearing."

People were chuckling now.

"I'M SORRY!" This time, he said it loud and clear.

With that, I winked at his girlfriend and told her she could do a lot better than this asshole, and walked back to the counter. At the till the cashier was looking at me with wide eyes.

Leaning forward, she said quietly, "That was the coolest thing I have ever seen."

I chuckled and paid for my Ice Cappuccino, and left.

"Henry owes me one!"

Sometimes being muscular can lead to situations that can take you totally by surprise. On one particular occasion, I was at a sales call at an elderly couple's house. It was my job to see if they needed a new furnace, which they did as their current one was 40 years old and clearly on its last legs. If memory serves me right, the woman's name was Betty, and the gentleman's name was Henry. She was 78, and he was 82 years old. They were very pleasant to deal with and quite sweet.

After I had wrapped up the paperwork and was about to leave, Betty quietly said, "May I ask one small favour of you, Todd?"

I answered, "Yes, of course."

I still can't believe what happened next.

She asked, "Can I feel the muscle in your arm, please?"

I felt my cheeks get warm as I walked over to Betty as she motioned for me to flex my bicep. As I did so, she grabbed my arm with both of her hands and exclaimed, "Oh my!" Then she looked over at Henry, her voice taking on a serious tone she remarked, "Henry, you're going to get lucky tonight!"

I looked over at Henry as a big wide smile crossed his lips as he was nodding his head in approval.

We all laughed, and I said, "Have fun, you two, and Henry, you owe me one!"

"Hey yo, Herculeeeez!"

Sometimes being big and muscular can have its advantages. I was in St. Louis for a sales training course and was staying in a downtown hotel. In my off hours, it was important to find a gym as I was not far out from a competition, so missing workouts was not an option. When visiting other towns, I also like to train in gyms I might otherwise not get to. Luckily enough, the front desk clerk directed me to a gym about a mile away from the hotel.

It was mid-evening as I started out. Before I got to the front doors of the hotel, the clerk asked me, "Sir, it's getting late. Do you feel ok walking around downtown by yourself?"

Being a hot day, I was already in my gym attire, a Gold's Gym tank top and sweats. I gave her a look that must have said, "You ARE kidding, right?"

As she looked me up and down, she laughed and said, "Never mind, yeah, I think you will be ok."

I headed down the street, carrying my gym bag, and I was in quite a good mood. I was enjoying St. Louis. Sometimes, it's just nice to get away, even if I had to sit through a boring sales course all day.

As I was walking along, I noticed that I seemed to be the only white person in the entire downtown area. Being from a large multicultural city in Canada, I had never been in a situation where I was the only white guy around. It didn't bother me. It was just something that occurred to me.

It was as I was crossing a side street that I heard a voice call out, "Hey yo, check it out. YO YO YO, hey man! Hey yo, Herculeeeez!"

Without turning my head, I could see through my peripheral vision that there were about five young African American men all hanging out by a car listening to music. Downtown Winnipeg could be a scary place at night, so I did as I always would do back home. I kept looking straight ahead and continued on my way.

He called out a second time, "Yo man! Yo, I said hey, you in the TANK TOP!"

He really exaggerated the words "tank top." It was pretty obvious he was talking to me. I stopped. Now I had a decision to make, "Five against one. Not good." was my thought. Running was not my modus operandi, so I put my gym bag down and turned as slowly and as ominously as I could.

"Look big!" was the thought that ran through my head. I looked at them like I wanted them all dead and shouted back, "WHAT?!?"

The young man looked at me and struck a "Which way to the beach" muscle pose as he yelled out, "Hey brother, give me one of these!" With that, his whole crew busted out laughing. I couldn't hold it in. The way he said it was so animated that I cracked and started laughing as well. The tension was broken, and I hit the same pose.

After that, I walked over to them, and we shared some laughs as they asked me various questions about training and food. Every day that I was in St. Louis, I would walk by that street on my way to the gym. They were there every night. Without fail, they would call out, "It's the Canadian Herculeeeez!" Sometimes, being big is good!

"A star is born."

Many Canadian cities are used in the film and television industry as it is often more cost-effective to film in Canada than in the United States. Winnipeg is utilized a lot as many areas of the city can be disguised as large American cities. On a whim, I decided to go out for an open casting call. Before you knew it, I was getting small extra roles in some of these productions. Usually, if they needed someone to play a bouncer, or bartender, or bodyguard, I would get the call.

On one occasion, I got a call to be an extra on a low-budget film that Patrick Swayze and his wife were producing. It was a dance movie, and I was simply a background extra in a coffee shop/bookstore in Winnipeg's trendy exchange district. On set, there is a lot of downtime as camera angles are set up as well as lighting and so forth. Most of the time is spent waiting around until it is time to shoot. Mr. Swayze was decent to everyone on set. He even had his dog with him; an African breed called a Rhodesian Ridgeback.

I remember thinking, "what a great guy. He's this big star and so nice to everyone. Even has his dog here!"

In between takes, I was talking to another extra, and unbeknownst to me, Patrick Swayze was standing directly behind me. When the Assistant Director called for us to return to our "places," I turned around quickly and, in my exuberance, I knocked Mr. Swayze right on his ass! I stood over him with my mouth open like an idiot. He wasn't a big man, despite looking quite heroic onscreen. He was a little shorter than I and probably 60 or more pounds lighter. Very trim. Finally, as he looked up at me, he reached up his hand for me to help him to his feet, which I quickly did. In fact, I pulled him a little TOO hard and almost made him wipe out a second time.

I figured, "I'm done. I just knocked over the star. They are going to send me home!"

I felt really stupid as I started to stutter out an apology, "Mr. Swayze, I'm so sorry!"

He just smiled and laughed, "Calm down, it's ok. No harm, no foul. Just be careful. You're kind of a big fella!" As he said this, he patted me on the chest.

For the rest of the shoot, all I kept thinking was, "Geez, I knocked Patrick Swayze on his ass!"

There is good, and there is bad. One thing I know for sure when you live your life as a bodybuilder, it's going to be different!

CHAPTER 34

Prelude to Cookie Dough

Hindsight is indeed 20/20. Perhaps it is normal for most of us to look back upon our lives and think, "If only I knew then, what I know now!" This is certainly the case for me. Another saying that I often hear in the bodybuilding world is, "Go big or go home!" Unfortunately, I applied that not only to my training and bodybuilding, I also applied it to my course of self-destruction. Deep down, on a subconscious level, I knew what I was doing. I knew that I was destroying myself. Sadly, it didn't matter. My life was still training, living with Denise, and seeing Aubrey. Most of the time, I did not feel much in the way of emotion. If I felt anything, it was usually anger. When I think back to this period in my life, the words "ticking time bomb" come to mind.

As I continued with my preparations for the upcoming bodybuilding season, I, of course, continued using various anabolic compounds to make sure that I brought the best possible total package to any shows I was entering. I was toying with the idea of competing Provincially even though I had already qualified for Nationals.

I thought it might be fun to compete in my hometown and that it would be a good tune-up for the bigger National event that was held a few weeks later. By this point, I did not give much thought to my use of steroids. It was part of bodybuilding and was, for the most part, an accepted part. The amounts I used were still considered on the "moderate" side, especially compared to the amounts I knew some of the other guys used. Still, I was using more than I ever had in the past. You never worry that something bad might happen until it does. My bout with pancreatitis seemed so long ago, and truthfully, I never thought anything could hurt me. I felt bulletproof.

The painful lump that began to grow on my right hip/upper glute area was the result of an injection. I thought nothing of it. After all, it was common on occasion to have some swelling or pain from intramuscular injections. "It will be gone in a few days." That was my thinking anyway. It did not go away. The lump started to become quite painful and was the size of a golf ball after about three days. I continued to ignore it and took no time off training. After all, I was invincible. I was limping from the pain, and yet, the thought of seeing a Doctor never entered my mind. It was business as usual, lump or no lump. Hindsight, sigh.

It was around 8:00 pm one Friday evening when I received a panicked text from Aubrey. Her roommate John was drunk and possibly high as well and was threatening her. This was happening in front of her young daughter and her daughter's friend that was there for a sleepover. He was behind in rent, and she had suspicions that he was stealing from her as well. When she confronted him about the rent, he lost it. She was scared and texted me for help.

I know you're thinking, "Why didn't she call the police?"

Well, Aubrey lived in a rough part of town, and her experiences with the police had not been favourable. In fact, the couple times she had to call them in the past, all she received for her troubles were cops hitting on her.

"Keep him there!" I instructed as I headed out to my car. I told Denise what was going on and where I was going. Denise knew about Aubrey, well, kind of. She thought I was just training her. She obviously did not know that I was seeing her as well.

The drive to Aubrey's house would normally take 20-30 minutes, depending on traffic. I was there in less than 15. When I arrived, John was outside of Aubrey's house, leaning on his girlfriend's car.

As a child, I had witnessed my mother taking a beating from one of her brothers. I was terrified and angry, and there was nothing I could do as a small boy. During the drive over, that memory had resurfaced, and I was getting madder with each passing second. I was no longer a little boy, no longer helpless. If there was one thing that angered me more than anything, it was a man threatening or beating a woman.

I came screeching to a halt next to where John was standing. Once out of my car, I could see John's eyes grow wide with fear. As I started walking towards him, he started to talk extremely fast, "T-ttodd, it's ok, we worked it out, its o—"

I didn't let him finish. I picked him up by his shirt collar until his feet were off the ground. He let out a yelp. John was an average-sized man, about 6 ft tall and maybe 170lbs. I didn't care. I was enraged. I slammed him into his girlfriend's car and watched him slump to the ground.

Reaching down, I lifted him to his feet and then elevated him a second time. I then slammed him down onto the hood of my car. I held him in place with one hand and pulled my right arm back as though I was about to punch him in the face.

He started to beg, "Please, Todd, I'm sorry, please don't!"

I growled at him, "Do you know who the fuck I am? I'm Aubrey's fucking boyfriend! You threaten to beat her up in front of her kid!?! What the fuck is wrong with you?!? You want to beat up a woman? You don't seem so fucking tough now!!!"

He continued to beg and plead with me not to hit him as his girlfriend was yelling in the background. Not about what I was doing to John, but that I had dented her car when I threw him into it.

"Nice woman you got there, John!" I remember thinking.

I picked him up off the hood of my car and slammed him to the pavement. This time, knocking the wind out of him. It had taken a lot of self-control to not smash his face in as all my anger was spilling out of me. I lifted him up, holding him by his shirt, and began to explain to him what was going to happen next, "You're leaving tonight, John. You are packing up your shit and moving out. You are going to pay Aubrey what you owe her, and then you are never coming back. IF you come back or contact her in any way, I will find you. Do you understand?"

He nodded and asked, "Can I get some friends to help me move my stuff?"

"NO! You can bring one person to help you. If either of you even looks at me or tries anything stupid, I will cave both of your faces in!" I let him go and started to walk towards Aubrey's house. His girlfriend was still squealing about her dented car. I couldn't resist, "Nice girlfriend, you got there, buddy! Real caring. She's a keeper!"

With that, I walked into the house to make sure Aubrey and her daughter were ok. She thanked me, and I explained that John would be leaving that night. I then grabbed a baseball bat that Aubrey had and sat and waited for John and his buddy to return to collect his things. When they arrived, I sat in a chair watching them, baseball bat across my lap. They did not look at me once. John gave me the money he owed for rent, and that was it. They were gone.

After the dust had settled, I became aware that I was in extreme pain—the lump. Throwing John around had aggravated it.

Aubrey looked at me and asked, "Are you ok?"

Something wasn't right. I was sweating profusely, and the pain was intensifying.

"Yeah, I'm good." I kissed her goodbye and told her that I would return should John come back. All she had to do was let me know if he did. I hid my limp as I walked to my car. When I got home, Denise asked me what happened. I explained that I evicted her roommate, leaving out some of the details.

Denise could not understand why I did what I did. "It's not your problem, Todd!"

My response was to the point, "Single Mom, being threatened. I had no choice!"

Denise had a bad feeling about the whole situation, and she made it clear. She did not like it one bit. I started to limp off to bed, and she asked, "Why are you limping?" I could no longer hide it. The pain was intense. I made up something about a slight muscle pull in my hip and went to bed.

The next morning the golf ball-sized lump had grown into a baseball-sized one. I was pretty sure it was an abscess caused by my last injection. I had experienced them in the past but never to this degree. Still, I continued to lie to myself and went about my daily routine as if there was nothing wrong.

"Are you sure you can train? You're not moving very well." I could hear the concern in Denise's voice. I waved it off, and we drove to the gym and worked out. By that evening, I had to admit that it was time to go to the hospital. The lump was now the size of a softball, and I could barely walk. Denise helped me to the car, and off we went.

"You want to do what!?!" I could not believe what the Doctor was saying. I was right; it WAS an abscess and a severe one at that. However, the thought of him slicing me open with no anesthetic would be bad enough under ordinary circumstances. Never mind that the lump was so painful to the touch I could no longer even sit down. The second option was a huge dose of antibiotics. The likelihood of the drugs even making a dent in the infection was unlikely, to say the least, as it was too late in the game. I still chose option two and returned home, hoping for an overnight miracle. The next morning it was even worse, and I knew I had no choice but to return to the hospital and get the lump cut out.

To say that the procedure was painful is a very large understatement. It was an awful, bloody mess. After the Doctor was finished, he sutured me up and sent me on my way with a prescription for pain meds.

Once home, I was so exhausted. I fell asleep almost immediately.

A couple of hours later, I woke up to go to the bathroom and noticed a strange sensation on my leg. I was wet, soaking wet. I called Denise into the room to look, and she quickly discovered I was bleeding badly through the dressing. She changed the bandage, and once finished, she brought me some pain meds that I used to dose myself into oblivion.

When I woke up not an hour later, I was shocked to find that I had once again bled through the dressing. When we saw how much blood there was, we knew we had to return to the hospital. Once there, we were instructed to sit and wait for an available Doctor.

After about ten minutes, I heard Denise let out an audible gasp, "Todd, look down."

I was sitting in a pool of my own blood. I was bleeding out at an alarming rate.

"Fuck me!" I thought as I got to my feet and staggered to the nurse at the triage station.

She was helping a young lady that had what looked to be a small wound on her head. However, she was acting quite dramatic as her boyfriend was comforting her.

"Sorry to interrupt," I began, "I think I need some help!"

The boyfriend turned his head and was starting to say something like, "Wait your turn...." when he spied the large trail of blood that led to the pool of it that had collected under the chair I had been sitting on. He didn't say another word. They admitted me right away and did their best to stop the bleeding.

Apparently, the Doctor I had seen was not a surgeon, and he had completely botched the procedure. I was rushed to another hospital where they had a surgeon that was available to help. I was rushed into surgery quite quickly, and this time, they got it right. The experience was not over yet. As the wound was left opened and packed. It would have to heal slowly over time, with me making many trips to an outpatient clinic to have the dressing repackaged as it healed.

Sometimes if it didn't look like it was healing well, they would chemically cauterize it. I still remember the terrible pain and the smell of my flesh as it burned.

A normal person would perhaps take a step back to rethink everything. Not me. Within a few days, I was back in the gym training. Usually, with extra bandages and dressing on hand in case I started to bleed, which happened more often than not. Despite everything, I was determined to win Nationals and turn pro.

The knock on the front door came as a complete surprise to me. Almost no one even knew where I lived, and I liked it that way. Denise was at work, so it was unlikely that it could be one of her family members. When I answered the door, I was greeted by two plainclothes police officers. The next thing I knew, I was being led away in cuffs. John had pressed assault charges against me. Or rather, his girlfriend MADE him press assault charges. Thankfully, the officers let me text Denise to let her know what was going on.

On the drive to the police station, the two officers asked me various questions about training and food. They were trying their very best to befriend me, it seemed. Like somehow, I was going to forget that I was handcuffed and in the back of an unmarked police cruiser.

"So, I hear bodybuilders can pretty much get their hands on any steroid or drug they want. Is that true?" he asked me like we were long-lost buddies.

I answered him bluntly, "Bodybuilders? I'm quite sure that these days anyone can get any drug they want if they ask enough people."

It almost seemed like he was waiting for me to say, "Steroids? Sure, I can get you some. What do you need?" It was comical. Once down at the station, I was placed into an interrogation room, and they got down to business. I simply and politely replied I had no interest in giving a statement until I spoke with my attorney.

They did not give up easily and listed off a long list of injuries that John "supposedly" had as a result of me punching and kicking him. Which, of course, was not what happened.

Finally, I decided to say one thing to them, "Have you fellows met John?"

They both assured me they had.

"Ok," I said, "and now you are sitting here looking at me." I continued, "Did John have any marks or bruises on his face where I supposedly hit him?"

They both stated that he had no marks on him.

"Ok, so guys, if I punched either one of you in the face even once, don't you think there might be a mark?"

They both laughed at that, and I was proud of my little "Perry Mason" moment. I was released later that day with a bunch of paperwork and a court date. I wasn't overly affected by the whole incident. Like always, my focus was on my training, and this little "issue" was more of a nuisance than anything.

Not caring, as in, "I do not have one fuck to give!" is possibly the worst state of mind to be in. So, when my "friend" asked me to pick up another package from Calgary, my reply was, "Sure, why not?" I was about two weeks away from competing in the Provincial Bodybuilding Championships, and I decided to once again drive to Calgary.

I thought, "This time, I will bring Denise, let her see Gold's Gym and the city, and maybe convince her that moving there would be beneficial to us." Even though I was still seeing Aubrey, although that had cooled somewhat after my arrest, I thought Denise would make a great partner. We decided to put the dogs in a kennel and drive out for a couple of days.

At the last minute, Denise came down with a terrible cold. I decided to go anyway. I wanted to hit Gold's, train there, and talk to them a little more seriously about a job. The trip was uneventful other than I had pretty much decided that a move to Calgary was a great option. Of course, things became a little more eventful when I was not even a block from my house, and I was pulled over by five cop cars and had a gun pointed at my head!!!

This time around, however, I wasn't quite so cocky on the ride to the Police station. I kept thinking about what the one Officer said to me after I had been cuffed and thrown in the back of his cruiser, "I bet it ain't cookie dough!"

As we drove in silence, I kept thinking, "Why didn't I ask what was in the package? I'm not an idiot. Yet, I had agreed to pick up a package for someone that I really didn't know that well. Was it because the last time it was just cell phones? Then again, I didn't ask last time either. So why didn't I ask?" I felt numb. Not scared. Not worried. Numb. Then it came to me, the answer:

I didn't care.

CHAPTER 35

Self-fulfilling Prophecy

A good friend of mine once told me something that I believe to be true. That is, "Some people are prophetic." It was his belief that in some instances, people might have dreams or thoughts that were a glimpse into future events. I personally do not believe that I am gifted in that regard, with one exception. Ever since I was a child, I could clearly envision myself in prison. Whenever I would watch a movie or TV show that dealt with prisons or people being incarcerated, I would think about how I was going to conduct myself WHEN I went to jail. Notice I said when and not if. I simply could see it, which was a little weird as I had led a very clean and law-abiding life right up until the incident that led to my assault charge.

As I was led into a holding cell, I was starting to come to the realization that I was probably not going home anytime soon. After a few minutes, the arresting officers entered and sat down in front of me. I do not remember their names, but I do remember that they were very professional in every way.

After the interview (with me explaining that I had nothing to say without my attorney being present), they even brought me a couple of protein bars to eat. I was processed and fingerprinted and then led back to the holding cell. I was exhausted.

When the officers finally returned, I had one question for them, "What was in the package?"

I think it was only then that they realized that I really didn't know. "Crystal meth. Probably over $50,000.00 worth."

My heart sank as I thought, "I am truly fucked."

I was then handed over to a couple of uniformed constables for transport. They not only handcuffed me, but they also shackled me at the ankles as well. Then they asked the question that I was going to be asked many more times before my ordeal was over, "You're not going to give us any problems, are you?"

To which I gave what was to become my standard reply, "No. I'm fine."

Police officers (and correctional officers) have an almost impossible job to begin with, and I think that asking that question was a way for them to ascertain if I was going to give them any grief. They always seemed relieved when they saw that I was cooperating, and often the tension would be broken with a joke from either them or myself. The way I looked at it, the situation was already horrible. Why make it worse?

After I answered, one of the constables joked, "Thank God! You are the last guy I want to have a problem with!"

I was being transported to the Remand Centre, which is a pre-trial detention centre located in Downtown Winnipeg. During the drive, the constables made small talk with me about the usual training and what they should eat to lose weight. I was still in shock. I had been allowed to call Denise and explain what happened and tried to comfort her best as I could.

I told her, "Don't worry, I will be home soon."

Of course, I had no idea when I would be going home, if at all.

Once at the Remand, I was processed and then ordered to strip down. I was searched and ordered to bend over and spread my butt cheeks so they could see that I was not trying to sneak anything into the detention centre. I was then ordered to shower and was given an orange jumpsuit to wear.

From there, I was escorted by a female officer to an elevator that would take me to my new "home." Once in the elevator, the guard started to chuckle. She stopped herself, and then the giggling started again.

I could not hold back from asking, "I fail to see the humour in this situation. Do you mind telling me what's so damn funny?

Her answer gave me a small modicum of relief, "I was just thinking, you have nothing to worry about!"

At first, however, I didn't understand, so I asked, "What do you mean?"

She continued, "You look concerned. Look at the size of you. No one is going to bother you, don't worry!"

Inside I let out a sigh of relief. After all, until you have been incarcerated, you really do not know what to expect. Movies and TV tend to sensationalize prison. There are, at least, some inherent truths to what the entertainment business would have you believe. They just tend to exaggerate. For the most part, the inmates I met would try to avoid unnecessary hassles.

As it turns out, the correctional officer was right. Not only did I not get bothered, no one even spoke to me for the first three days I was there. Finally, on day four, I was sitting by myself during one of the brief respites that were given to us from our cells. A young man in his early twenties sat down next to me and said, "Um, can I ask you a question?"

Without looking in his direction, I nodded.

"Are you getting enough to eat in here? I mean, you probably eat a lot of fuckin food!"

I looked at him and quietly said, "No. I'm not."

With that, he got up and quickly walked away. When he returned, he handed me three packs of instant oatmeal, "Here, man, you need this more than I do."

I was shocked and tried to refuse it, "Keep your food, bro."

He was insistent. Friends and family can buy inmates items from the canteen, including food items. I was amazed at this fellow's act of kindness.

Then he asked, "Can you tell me how to get arms like yours?"

I could not help but laugh. Here we were, locked up in prison, and still, I was being asked about training and bodybuilding. I guess that broke the ice, and gradually the other inmates started to talk to me. One lent me some Muscle Magazines to read, and I was no longer eating my meals by myself.

A common question that they asked me was, what had I done to end up in here. When I told them, they were very blunt in their responses. It was usually something like, "Meth!?! Fuck no, bro. That sucks, bro! You are going away for a looooong time!" I hated that conversation every time it came up.

Something else I had not considered when I first got to the Remand was the fact that I would know some of the correctional officers, and some of them would recognize me from bodybuilding. To say that was awkward is an understatement. In fact, one of the guards had been a boyfriend of one of Mandy's friends and had been to our house on more than one occasion.

Not wanting to make things worse for me, he waited until he had a chance to talk to me with no other inmates around to hear. It was more than embarrassing to explain what had happened. There were some advantages however, whenever there was any extra food at mealtimes, the officers would always offer it to me. I always took it. The last thing I wanted to do was waste away while locked up. I exercised in my cell as we were not allowed access to the weight room very often.

On the fifth day, they gathered up a group of us and brought us to an elevator that would bring us down to the exercise facility. I was anxious to train with weights as this had been the longest training hiatus that I had in quite some time.

Once in the elevator, the largest inmate said to me, "Hey, big fucker. What would you do if I shoved you right now?"

I answered in the best "Arnold" accent I could muster, "You only get the one-shot, then I put you through the Goddamn wall!!!"

Everyone in the elevator erupted in laughter, including the big fellow. The tension was broken. Once in the exercise facility, I felt a tiny bit of peace for the first time since I had arrived. Many of the inmates simply stood around and watched to see how much I could lift. That was flattering in its own way.

Any chance of my arrest going unnoticed by the local bodybuilding community was lost simply due to the fact that I knew more than a few of the guards that worked at the Remand. Even though the Officers are not supposed to talk about the identities of those incarcerated, it was inevitable that people would find out.

My lawyer was doing his best to get me out, and in the meantime, all I could do was sit and wait as my reputation was destroyed. The story that was circulating was that I was a connected meth dealer. Even though I had more than enough time to think about how bad my situation was, my survival instincts had kicked in. I didn't have time to be depressed. I had to find a way out. I was going to miss competing at Provincials, which sucked. That wasn't my goal, though; it was a warmup for Nationals. Even though I was in prison, and my life was shattering all around me, I still held on to the insane notion that winning the National Championship would fix EVERYTHING! I was delusional, to say the least.

After about a week at the Remand, I was transferred to Milner Ridge Correctional Centre, located in rural Manitoba. I was shackled and put into the back of a van to be transported to my new digs. It was two other inmates and me. We were seated on metal benches with no seatbelts of any kind. It did not make for a comfortable trip. All I kept thinking was, "Please God, do not let us get into an accident!" Seeing as we were basically riding along in a steel box, I was quite sure that any accident would result in grievous injuries or death.

Once at Milner, I was asked the standard, "You're not going to give us any trouble, are you?"

I was then processed and led to my cell that was in a unit that housed individuals affiliated with gangs. I was only allowed out of my cell for one hour a day. My lawyer had advised me that I needed to find someone that could sign a surety for me. That is, an individual that would put themselves on the line to ensure that I would not try and take off before my trial, should I be released from prison. This is usually done by allowing a lien to be placed on your house. So, if I skipped town or breached any conditions or curfews that were placed on me, the surety would be on the hook for it! I called EVERYONE that I knew and considered a friend. Not surprisingly, no one would take that kind of risk to set me free. After all, I was a meth dealer in everyone's eyes!

I trained as best as I could, performing only bodyweight exercises. For some reason, I clung to the hope that I would be released and vindicated. Nationals was still my goal. Each day that passed saw me falling into a darker and deeper depression. One does not really know what freedom is until you have had it taken away. What made it worse was that I was in prison because of my own stupidity and foolish actions. I had no one to blame but myself and those thoughts would haunt me every moment I was awake and sometimes in my dreams.

Every day I called Denise until the inevitable happened. Denise and Aubrey had been talking since my arrest. In time, Denise started to wonder why Aubrey seemed to care so much about my situation, and she flat out asked Aubrey if we were having an affair. Aubrey admitted to her that yes, we were together.

As you can imagine, the next call to Denise did not go very well. She had every right to be angry. I had put her through hell, embarrassed her. To top it all off, she now found out that the man she loved was cheating on her. I felt horrible.

The only silver lining was that she could now break away from the horrible situation of her boyfriend being incarcerated, and there would be no one that would blame her in any way for leaving me! She deserved better. Denise was and is a good person. It was going to get way worse, and I was relieved that she would be spared all of it.

The next time I was permitted to use the phone, I called Aubrey and asked her, "Why Aubrey? Why did you tell her?"

Her explanation was simple enough, "It was wrong. I couldn't lie anymore."

She had done the right thing. Through it all, Aubrey was the only person that stuck by me at all. Everyone else in my life basically washed their collective hands of me.

Each day that passed by, I found myself sinking a little deeper into a black hole of despair. Having so much time to think did not help matters. Then I heard it. A quiet little voice came to me in my slumber one morning after breakfast. I was lying on my bunk, having dozed off, but there it was in my head.

Coach K's voice, "Shoulder down, Todd! Drive the lane!"

I was back in my high school gym, playing ball against Steven Sacher. I put my shoulder down and drove to the hoop! Layup. Then I was back at the foul line, ready to go again, only this time it wasn't Steven I was playing against. It was my biological father. He was scowling at me. I tried to drive past him, but he knocked me down.

I got up and looked over at Coach K as he said, "You got this, don't give up!" I tried again. BAM! I hit the floor with force.

Neil was laughing now. I got up. Feeling tears well up in my eyes, I looked at Coach. Then I had an epiphany. I'm not 12 years old anymore! I'm grown, and I'm strong. My body changed into myself as an adult. I took the ball, drove through my father, and scored.

I woke up with tears rolling down my cheeks. I was angry with myself. This was NOT how I was going to go out! I started to change my outlook. I refused to believe that I was going to stay in prison. Then something else happened. I prayed. For the first time in many years, I prayed to God and asked Him for strength.

The next time I called Aubrey, I asked her a very tough question, "Aubrey, will you be my surety?"

I explained what was involved, how she would have to let them put a lien against her house, and that if I screwed up, she would be on the hook for $50,000.00. To my surprise, she agreed to do it. I am not sure if she felt some guilt because of our affair or my arrest because of the incident with John, but she did it.

It took a few days for everything to be processed, and then it happened. I was released. I had been locked up for five weeks in total. Not very long, really. However, it was the longest five weeks of my life! Before I walked out of the gate, the correctional officer that was escorting me shook my hand and said, "I really hope I never see you back here. You don't belong in prison."

I thanked him and assured him it would never happen again if I had any say in the matter. There was Aubrey, standing outside of her car, looking amazing. I walked up to her and hugged her harder than I had ever hugged anyone in my life. It felt amazing to be outside again and free. Well, somewhat free. I had conditions and curfews. Compared to being locked up, it was a cakewalk.

I don't remember much about the drive. In fact, I am pretty sure I had a little blackout. Aubrey drove me back to the house that I had been renting with Denise. The rent had been paid from money that Denise had collected from the sale of my furniture. It was the last thing that Denise had done for me. My landlord was evicting me after that month was up. The police had searched the house right after my arrest, and he was notified. He wanted no part of a "drug dealer" living in his rental property.

Reality set in after Aubrey had dropped me off. Once inside the house, I began to crack up. My momentary strength had vanished. The house was completely empty. Denise had the dogs. The power had been shut off. I had running water, but only cold.

I started to walk from room to room. It hit me like a ton of bricks. I had no job, no money, no food, and I was totally alone. For the very first time in my life, I felt finished. I had been down before. This time was different. I felt empty inside. I had been good at finding a way to get through challenges in my life. This was the first time that I really had no idea where to start.

I kept wandering from room to room, then I saw it in the bathroom. Painkillers. They were left over from my accident. I took them in my hand and kept walking and pacing. It felt hopeless—the situation, my life. The demons were winning. This was it. Bottom. Had the dogs been there, had anyone been there, I would not have taken the pills. But I was alone. I had enough. I did not blame a single person for where I was at. I put myself there. Perhaps that was the hardest part to deal with.

I sat on the kitchen floor and said what I thought would be my final prayer.

Down went the pills. I felt myself getting sleepy. As far as I was concerned, I was finished. God, however, had a different plan for me.

CHAPTER 36

Total Rebuild

It was a loud knocking on the door that woke me up. "Todd! Are you there? Todd, open the door!"

It was Aubrey. I woke up feeling quite groggy. I was confused. Dizzy. I staggered to the door and opened it. There stood Aubrey, bags of food in hand.

"You look like shit!" was her greeting.

"I feel like shit."

She walked in and placed the bags of food on the kitchen counter, "It's not much, but I brought you some tuna and some other things…" her voice trailed off when she noticed the empty pill bottle. "How many of these did you take?"

I mumbled, "I don't know, whatever was left."

It was all coming back to me now. I had wanted to die. Apparently, there were not enough pills to kill me, just more than enough to knock me senseless.

"Denise and I figured you might do that," she said flatly.

"Sorry to disappoint you both. I'm still here."

Aubrey just laughed at that. She had brought some protein powder, and I made myself a shake and quickly drank it. She asked me what I wanted to do or if I needed to go anywhere.

Then it came to me, "The gym, take me to the gym."

"How will you get back?" she inquired.

"I will walk. I could use a good walk."

When I entered the gym, I immediately saw some other competitors. Normally, I would walk over and say, "Hi.". When they saw me, they not only got quiet, but they also literally turned their backs towards me.

"So, this is how it's going to be, huh?" was all I could think.

A strange thing happened next. I felt calm. Peace. My mind turned off as I started to train. Bench press. Good old bench press. My muscles started to warm up as I added weight to the barbell with each progressive set. 225lbs, 275lbs, 315lbs, it still felt good.

I decided to keep increasing the weight—365lbs and then finally 405lbs.

Normally, I would have someone spot me at that much weight. If something goes wrong with 405lbs over your chest, it could be a disaster! I felt like a leper. No one was going to help, "Fuck it! I will do it anyway." I lifted the weight off the rack and performed six smooth reps, and then slammed it back onto the supports. I felt a wave of relief. I was still strong.

Just then, I saw a fellow named Jay I knew from competitions. He walked over and said, "Todd, hey. How are you, man? I heard some things. Everything ok?"

He was the only one decent enough to talk to me.

"Well, Jay, I will put it this way…some of the stuff you have heard is probably true. Some is probably bullshit. I'm here, training. Still benching over 400lbs. So maybe, things are not as bad as people are saying!"

I'm not sure if I said that for his benefit or my own. Still, it was nice that he came and said, "Hi." He was the only one.

I started to take mental ownership of the situation. I had to admit to myself that even though I had truly hit rock bottom, I WAS still here, still alive. No matter how shitty this situation was, many people had it much worse. It was time to pull my head out of my ass and get on with it. So, I had to figure out what assets I had left.

As far as I could tell, I had three things, well, four really. I had my health (other than the passing out thing, which I could control to a degree), I had the ability to communicate well, I had a friend in Aubrey, and I had God. I realized while I was locked up that I needed to believe in something larger than myself. So, I had started talking to God. As far as Christians go, I pretty much sucked at being one. However, I felt that praying to God would not hurt!

I needed a plan that went beyond the thought of competing at Nationals. Survival became the first obstacle to tackle. I needed a job. I decided to go back to the Volkswagen dealership that I had worked at in the past. They were surprised to see me. I kicked it into high gear and sold them on the idea of hiring me back. This took some real salesmanship, but I won them over.

I wasted no time. The first day I worked, I sold three cars. I finished the month number one in the store. It was good to get a paycheque.

In the meantime, I was quite literally living on hot dogs with no buns and boloney and some eggs as well. Basically, the cheapest protein I could find. It felt very much like the days of being homeless. On more than one occasion, I had to resist the urge to steal food.

Instead, I focused on my job. I still went to the gym, but the workouts were brief. Hot dogs and boloney didn't give one much in the way of energy, and I did not want to find myself losing any more muscle than necessary. At this point, my training was more for mental health than anything else. I am quite sure that without the endorphin release from lifting weights, I would have lost it. The gym was still my sanity during a time of total instability!

Each day was a challenge. My reputation had been destroyed. I decided to focus on daily goals. Very simple goals like, wake up, shower, go to work, work hard, go to the gym. I was breaking it down to the ridiculously simple. If I started thinking about everything I had been through, my brain would short circuit, and I would spiral down. Having been at the bottom, I had no desire to return there. Aubrey and I continued to see each other. Where our relationship had been mostly a physical one before, we had started to bond. We became a couple.

I thanked her every day for taking the risk that she did to have me released from prison. Not only that, but she also allowed me to move into her house as my landlord was only letting me stay in my place until the end of that month. Our relationship had a very interesting dynamic. We were either laughing our asses off together or ready to kill each other. We both had dominant personalities, and neither one of us would back down. Together we lived in a virtual zoo as a blended family of pets. Eventually, the total was four cats and five dogs. Somehow, we made it work.

Just when I started to feel a little bit of the stress being lifted from my shoulders, the bottom fell out. I was at work when a courier came and served me with the papers that would change the course of my life at that time. I could not believe what I read. Could this be real? The Provincial Bodybuilding Federation that I competed for had indefinitely suspended me because of my arrest. Today, I understand why.

At the time, I was livid! Bodybuilding had enough of an image problem. What our federation did NOT need was the media questioning them about one of their champions being arrested for transporting meth. I was losing what I loved the most. It had become my identity. I had to blame someone. There was no way I could come to grips with the thought that I had done it to myself.

I justified it, "I haven't been convicted! It's not my fault! How could they ban me when almost every competitor uses illegal drugs just to compete!"

I decided to fight the decision hard. I went to the media myself. I told my side of the story. It was the stupidest thing I could have done.

A week later, I lost my job. Even though I was leading the store in sales, they canned me. The reason was simple. They found out about my arrest. The general manager, Gerald, felt horrible letting me go. He genuinely liked me. It was a huge liability for them, though. I gave them the keys to my demo and walked home.

Telling Aubrey was the worst. We had started to make some headway, and now the carpet was pulled out from under us financially. Instead of giving up, instead of quitting on myself, I dug down deeper. I took a horrible job as a telemarketer that paid minimum wage. Still, it was better than staying at home and earning nothing.

I was going to crawl out of this. I was determined. After a few months, I managed to get a job as a welder. It was challenging as I still suffered from blackouts from time to time. Also, my lungs certainly did not appreciate all the smoke. The pay was substantially more, and it was certainly better than the alternative. Aubrey and I worked out together.

Competition or no, I was not going to let my body fall apart. Aubrey was naturally strong and had no problems pushing hard in the gym. Bodybuilding was helping me keep it together. Even though it was no longer the centre of my life. Instead, it had become a joyful activity. Seeing how hard I could train, pushing myself not to compete, but just as it had once been in my youth, something I simply loved!

Then there was the question of my impending trial. The prosecutors were seeking just under seven years in prison for yours truly. My lawyer wanted me to plead guilty and take a deal that would mean three years behind bars with the possibility of early parole. While I agreed that my actions were beyond stupid in associating with the people I did, not to mention not questioning the contents of the package. I could not fathom pleading guilty to the charges that were brought forth against me. I was not a drug dealer and would not plead guilty.

I decided that I needed a new lawyer. I went through four different lawyers over the course of almost six years until I found one who seemed to think there was a SLIGHT chance I could possibly avoid jail time.

Her name was Christine, and she was very patient and seemed to believe in me. That was exactly what I wanted: Hope. Living my life for that many years, not knowing if I was going to jail, was torturous, to say the least. It certainly took its toll on Aubrey and me. We did everything we could to make things work, but in the end, we would be better off as friends. We were together for five years in total.

I wish I could say that we parted on good terms, but we did not. Once again, that was my fault. I had met someone else. I ended things with Aubrey first and then moved on. She had done all she could for me, and I know that. She went above and beyond. No matter what we tried, we just could not make things work between us. Perhaps we were both too headstrong.

By this time, I had slowly made my way back into the bodybuilding world, not as a competitor but as a coach. I moved out of Aubrey's place and was renting a room in the house of a bodybuilder I knew. I brought one of my dogs, Pugsley. My blind little pug. He depended on me heavily, and to this day, the bond I have with this weird little dog is something I cherish a great deal!

I had still not had my day in court. Through it all, I had never stopped fighting. I had not given up. I realized that being a bodybuilding champion would not end my problems or deal with my demons. This was something I had to deal with myself. I had to deal with my mistakes and be accountable for everything I had done. This took more strength than I ever had to use in the gym. This was a daily and sometimes hourly battle.

When I could not do it alone, I would lean on God. I would pray. This was the time of my "Total Rebuild." I would not quit. I would not stop fighting. I would not die. My day in court was coming. I would have my chance to speak. It would be the biggest challenge of my life.

"Shoulder down!" Coach K would be right there with me, in spirit as he had always been.

CHAPTER 37

"But it ain't about how hard ya hit…"

For the first time in my life, I was going to live outside of Manitoba. It was a risk for sure, but one I was willing to take. I had been dating Leah for several months, and we were growing close. She happened to live in a small town in Saskatchewan, the neighboring province to Manitoba.

It was a five-hour drive from her small town of Melville to Winnipeg, and she made the trip as often as she could. She had a 4-year-old daughter named Lilly, so getting away wasn't that easy. Not to mention, I still had curfews that I had to adhere to and could not just come and go as I pleased.

We decided that to see if we had any shot at a future together, we needed to at least live in the same town. She really did not want to move her daughter to Winnipeg, so the decision was made to move to Saskatchewan.

My training business was once again keeping me busy after a very successful showing at the recent Novice Bodybuilding Championships. All my athletes placed in the top three of their respective classes except for one, and I felt he should have as well. One of my clients, Steve, was 67 years old and had Parkinson's disease. He placed 2nd in the Grandmaster category and won a special award for being the most inspirational athlete.

The local news had picked up his story, and it eventually made it to the National news as well. In a five-year period, I had gone from prison to being on our country's national news, and this time, not for breaking the law!

Moving was no easy task. I had to get permission from the court and pay a deposit as well. I was still waiting for my trial and would have to come back to Winnipeg for that. In the end, the court granted me permission to move, and before long, I was living in a tiny little house in a town that, in some ways, reminded me of Mayberry. I hadn't been there more than a couple of days when I heard a horse's hooves clip-clopping down the street. My house was located on Main street, and I looked out of my front window to indeed see a horse and buggy slowly passing by.

"Where the hell am I?" I thought in utter disbelief.

I had worked hard to rebuild my training business and now was watching it slowly fall apart. Winnipeg is a conservative city in some ways, and many of my clients did not like the thought of me training them online. They wanted that personal touch, meeting with me on a regular basis. I was getting by, but just barely. It was purely by chance that I realized that I could open my own business right here in town. My landlord had asked me if I might be interested in opening a gym in town. She had a commercial property that was going to be vacant and asked me if I might like to rent it. I assumed I could never afford it, not realizing that in a small town, rent was much more affordable.

As it turned out, her tenant stayed, and I lost out on that building. By that time, the wheels in my wee brain were already turning, and I decided that I would open a gym. When I told Leah of my plan, she looked at me like I was nuts. She was heavily into fitness and was planning on competing later that year for the first time. We had both dreamt of owning a gym, so full steam ahead it was. I utilized the savings I had and managed to find an investor to kick in enough money to purchase some very basic training equipment and weights. I am a big believer in basic training, so it was not necessary to have the latest and greatest.

Most of my equipment was used and very well-loved, and that suited us both just fine. We found a great property to rent right on Main street that the landlord would develop for us. It also had an apartment above it, and once finished, we would move in there as well.

Between the two of us, we came up with the name "IRONLION GYM," and we set about the task of setting up our little hardcore gym as soon as the building was ready. We opened on February 14th and were very relieved when people started to join and buy personal training sessions. For the first time in a long time, it felt as though things were coming together. I was even allowed to compete in the same bodybuilding show Leah was entering. Saskatchewan's bodybuilding federation could care less about my old charges and welcomed me with open arms. I no longer saw bodybuilding as my life's holy grail. Instead, I thought it might be an effective way to get exposure for our gym.

Alas, life has taught me that things are not always as they seem. For the most part, Leah and I got along well. However, there were times that her behaviour was erratic. She would lash out in anger. We developed trust issues as I had caught her in a couple of lies, which in turn made me act controlling and more like her father than her partner. I could not figure out why we were having these problems. I was undeterred, however, as I now had a lot invested in my new life here, so I pressed forward and did the best I could.

It was a very scary thing to start a new relationship and a business when there is a very real possibility that jail time could be in the cards in the immediate future. Leah was very aware of my legal situation. For the most part, it was the elephant in the room. We knew it was there but chose not to discuss it. Instead, we chose to believe that everything would work out and that somehow I would not be locked up for the next 6 or 7 years! I decided that I would think of only a positive outcome and did my absolute best to keep negative thoughts to a minimum. My court date was set for May of 2015, and time seemed to crawl very slowly as I literally was awaiting my day in court.

It was decided that I would travel to Winnipeg alone for my trial. Leah and I said goodbye like nothing unusual was happening. Neither one of us wanted to acknowledge that I might not be coming back. I would have no one there for moral support save one friend, Neoma.

I had dated Neoma briefly in high school. She attended the same private school as my friend Rob Kliewer. We had not seen each other in many years, and it was not until the funeral of Rob's father Bruno that we reconnected. We had a long talk after the funeral and decided to stay in touch.

Neoma had a very strong connection to God and her church, and when my life came crashing down, she was one of the few that offered moral support and guidance whenever I needed it. My relationship with God was strained at best. Neoma was often the one I turned to with questions and my feelings of unworthiness. She was my friend unconditionally, and I really feel that God was using her to help me. She offered to sit with me in court, and I am quite sure she prayed almost the entirety of my trial.

We have all seen various courtroom dramas on TV and in movies. Still, it is a very different feeling being the person on trial. I felt beyond helpless as the prosecuting attorney did her very best to make me look like a connected drug courier. It took everything in my power to keep my mouth shut as she gave her opinion of what had happened.

"That's not what happened!" I would whisper to Neoma. She would comfort me as best as she could as the prosecutor continued to attack my character and make me look like a criminal. When she interviewed the arresting officers, there was no mention of the fact that I had been punched in the face and thrown to the ground even though I had not resisted arrest. Still, I harboured no ill will to the two officers that took the stand, as neither one of them had struck me and had, in fact, treated me very well during the subsequent arrest and interrogation.

During a brief recess, I made a point of talking to them both. Asking them how they were doing and shaking their hands. I even joked with them about using two sets of handcuffs on me, "Did ya think I was going to turn green?!"

To which one of them replied, "Well, look at the size of you! I didn't want to take any chances!"

We had a good laugh, and I got the feeling that neither one of them wanted to see me in prison. They asked what I had been doing with my life and told them about IRONLION and Leah and her daughter.

When the court was back in session, I was finally asked to take the stand. The prosecutor did her absolute best to trip me up, confuse me, and get me to contradict myself. I was not worried as I felt that if I spoke the truth, it would all work out fine. Still, having someone try to rip you apart on the witness stand is beyond unsettling, and once again, I made sure to keep my composure. It was bad enough that I looked like a gorilla. I felt that I had to go above and beyond to show that I had made a horrible mistake and was not only aware of it but felt a tremendous amount of remorse. Things went a lot better when my attorney was asking the questions. I felt foolish admitting that I did not question the contents of the package and did my best to tell my side of the story.

Before the judge made her ruling, I could address the court. "This is it, Todd, if ever you were going to find the right words, now would be the time!" was my train of thought before I spoke.

I decided that it was best to be accountable, to not blame anyone but myself. I also pointed out how I had tried to rebuild my life, that I had not reoffended and was now contributing to society. I talked about

Leah and Lilly and our life together. I was close to tears, and it was not an act. It was as though so much of what had happened in my life was all coming to a head at that very moment. I thanked the court for allowing me to say my peace and sat down.

Waiting for the judge to return with her verdict was the most painstaking few minutes of my life. When she came back, she read the verdict, "Guilty of trafficking…."

I heard nothing after she said the word "GUILTY!"

My heart sank. She also found me guilty of having proceeds of a crime as I had been carrying several hundred dollars on me at the time of my arrest. Then the miracle occurred. Even though she found me guilty, she awarded me ZERO jail time and instead gave me house arrest and community service that would see me talking to youth groups about my experiences.

I could not believe it. I completely broke down. I cried like never before in my life.

After almost seven years of having this hanging over my head, it was over. I would have these legal conditions to contend with for two years less a day. Compared to almost seven years in jail, this was a gift!

I thanked God and my lawyer.

Neoma and I were in complete shock.

I called Leah with the good news. She seemed irritated that I had received house arrest.

This shocked me as I thought to myself, "It could have been much worse!"

I was going home a free man, kind of. I had never given up. I fought.

A quote from the latest Rocky movie (ROCKY BALBOA) kept going through my mind:

"Let me tell you something you already know. The world ain't all sunshine and rainbows. It's a very mean and nasty place, and I don't care how tough you are. It will beat you to your knees and keep you there permanently if you let it. You, me, or nobody is gonna hit as hard as life. But it ain't about how hard ya hit. It's about how hard you can get hit and keep moving forward. How much you can take and keep moving forward. That's how winning is done!"

CHAPTER 38

"It ain't over till it's over!"

Before I left Winnipeg after my trial, there were two things I had to do. First, I had to see my Mother. My arrest had been not only an embarrassment to our family but a tremendous strain on her emotionally. It was an amazing thing to be able to hug her and tell her that I was not going to prison.

Throughout everything, the thought of disappointing her after how she had literally sacrificed everything for me as a child weighed so heavily on my mind that it was often almost too much to bear. I told her that it was her example that she had set that kept me going. No matter how tough things were for my Mother, she never quit. That was something I got from her.

Neoma had once told me that she had never seen a person so unwilling to give up against impossible odds. My Mother was the living epitome of "SHOULDER DOWN!" I also visited my Father's gravesite. I sat by his tombstone and cleaned it off. I spoke to him. It felt like he was there. I thanked him for his sacrifice as well. In a sense, he had died so that I could live, not repeating his mistakes and falling down the well of alcoholism. I still love him and always will.

At this point, Leah and I were still running our little gym. We had our trials and tribulations as we helped each deal with our demons. In the subsequent months after my trial, I had learned why Leah's behaviour was, at times, erratic, to say the least. She was a drug addict.

I did not know it at the time, but when we met, she was trying desperately to break away from her addictions and pursue her dreams of competing as a bodybuilder. She had one foot in two completely different worlds. She relapsed hard, and we spent six months apart. After hearing how badly she was doing, I went to her.

When she opened the door of the little house she was renting, I barely recognized her. She was wasting away. Her muscular body was frail, and she looked exhausted. I did not know it that day, but she later admitted to me that she had hit bottom. She either wanted to die or to fight for her life. We talked and cried together. I asked her to come back to the gym to work out. I promised her I would close the gym to the public while we trained so she could do so without the eyes of our small community judging her. It killed me seeing this proud, strong woman so beaten down.

I only wanted to help. She decided to fight her demons and returned to the gym. She stopped her drug use with no help from anyone except the iron. Her body responded like nothing I had seen in 30 years of bodybuilding! She was gaining muscle back daily. She is one of the most genetically gifted bodybuilders I have ever seen in my life.

Now, without recreational drugs in her system, she developed at a geometric rate! I fully believe that if she continues to work towards it, she will turn professional. For the first time, we really talked and began to truly understand where we had both failed. We were better as friends. We still battle our demons. It's a process. I thank God every day for what I have in life. One day at a time, sometimes an hour at a time. You must keep moving forward. On some days, it's only an inch.

It's strange how things happen. I battled so hard for so long. I fought against myself. I certainly fought against my demons. I fought for my freedom, and I also fought so very hard for the right to return to Competitive Bodybuilding. When I finally realized that bodybuilding was not, in fact, my saviour or the cure all to life's problems, and when I had finally made peace with the fact that I may never step on stage again, well, that's when it happened.

Leah had been training for her second competition, the first since she had been drug-free. When a little voice spoke to me, "Wouldn't it be something if you could compete as well?"

On a whim, I contacted the President of the Saskatchewan Bodybuilding Federation and asked for permission to compete again. I had competed in two shows before the National Federation had found out I was competing again and subsequently suspended me indefinitely.

Our President suggested that I contact the Canadian Bodybuilding Federation and ask to be reinstated. She told me that Saskatchewan would back me 100%. Figuring I had nothing to lose, I emailed the National President.

To my surprise, a week later, the CBBF fully reinstated me. It was no longer my life's ambition to compete, and perhaps that is exactly why it happened when it did. I was now free to compete again. I had a complete paradigm shift. I could train and compete for the love of it, the artistry—for the reasons I had started training in the first place. It is a wonderful feeling knowing that once again, I might be able to grace the stage of the Mr. Canada Bodybuilding Competition.

I once again had the opportunity to present the body as art and to perform. There is a feeling of peace in my soul that never existed before. There is no pressure. It was no longer about winning a pro card. It's not about that. It's not even about me. Maybe what I do might move some people, maybe my story can show others that it is always worth fighting!

There will come a day when I will no longer take the stage. I could bow out gracefully now, whenever I chose to, on my terms—showing that no matter how dark your situation might be, there is light at the end of the tunnel. I've seen it. If everything I have been through helps ONE person, I can honestly say it was worth it.

Maybe it was Rocky Balboa that said, "It ain't over till it's over!" He was right. It wasn't over.

CHAPTER 39

It Only Took 30 Years!

"Number 107, please step forward. Number 107, step forward." I don't know how many times the emcee had called my number before I actually realized they meant me. I am quite sure it must have been more than once. After all, here I was, 30 years after reading "Arnold's Education of a Bodybuilder," standing on the stage of the prestigious NABBA Mr. Universe Competition in Birmingham, England. Now my number was being called out in the top six grouping at prejudging. Was this a dream? No. This was real. Very real, and I had just about killed myself to get there!

I suppose I should back up a bit. How in the world DID I get there?

My little gym was struggling. In all reality, it had been built for TWO trainers, not one. Even though Leah and I were on good terms, we were still training together after all. She had moved on to other things. Melville is a small town, and only so many people worked out with weights. Even fewer were willing to pay for personal training. My house arrest sentence was winding down, and I really had no ties to Melville other than my failing gym, which, like it or not, was a constant reminder of a failed relationship. I made the decision to sell my equipment at a loss and move on. Once I had served my sentence, I knew it was time to go. It had been my dream to move west, and now there was nothing standing in my way.

Calgary, Alberta. Truly a beautiful city. This would be where I would settle. I found a great gym, King's Fitness. It was the namesake of Leo King, a competitive powerlifter, bodybuilder, and promoter of bodybuilding competitions. This gym has everything one could ask for, including a "family" feel to it. Everyone supported one another, encouraged each other. In some ways, it reminded me of Olympik Gym. Leo's dog, "Kilo," was at the gym every day, and members were encouraged to bring their own dogs (as long as they were well behaved). Whenever I trained, I would invariably tune the music system to the AC/DC playlist, which I am quite sure many members grew tired of. Yet, nobody complained. They would often shake their heads and smile and sometimes make jokes about letting the "old guy" listen to his tunes. After all, at 49 years of age, I was technically "the old guy." I felt at home. My training intensity was the best it had been in years.

Being an "old guy" means that it is quite common to tell "old guy" stories. It was on one such occasion that I was recounting to one of my training partners that I had once received an invite to compete at the NABBA Mr. Universe competition. "If there was one contest I regret never competing in, that would be the one! Such history. It's where Arnold got his start." She looked at me like my elevator didn't go to the top floor as she stated in a very matter-of-fact fashion, "So, what's stopping you from trying again!?!"

That statement stopped me in my tracks. What did I have to lose? Nothing really. I mean, I was forever telling people that "you can't lose what you don't have!"

The first step was to speak to Si Sweeney. Si was and is an integral part of the NABBA organization. We had become long-distance friends via social media. Si knew my story, and in many ways, we shared similar experiences growing up. He was very supportive of the idea and suggested that I request an invitation to compete at the Universe as a representative of Canada.

He gave me Eddy Ellwood's email address and told me I should reach out to him. Eddy was a five-time Mr. Universe winner and an absolute bodybuilding legend. He was also on the executive committee of NABBA.

I was surprised at Eddy's quick response to my inquiry as he asked for some recent photos as well as my contest history. It was his job to make sure I was up to snuff. Canada did not have any qualifying contests for the Universe at the time, so it would be up to the executive to decide whether or not to invite me.

I was quite shocked at his reply email after I sent him everything he requested.

"You look good, Todd. I am going to forward your info to Val Charles, the NABBA president. I think you have a good chance at being invited."

Val Charles? She was the president when I had originally been invited to compete at the Universe. "Would she remember me?" was my first thought. Her email answered that exact question.

She wrote, "Well, Todd, it has taken a long time, but it looks like we will be getting you up on the Mr. Universe stage! Attached below is your official invitation and entry form. Best of luck in your preparations. Regards, Val Charles." I must have read that email a dozen times. I couldn't believe it. I was finally going to compete in the Mr. Universe competition.

The very first thing I did after receiving my invitation was to print it out and have it framed.

The second thing I did was to contact my friend Richard Politano. Richard was a former Mr. Universe competitor himself. He was trained by legendary coach Bob Gruskin. Bob was the original bodybuilding guru and trained more bodybuilding champions than anyone. Richard, a retired police officer, is a mountain of a man. Had he decided to seriously pursue bodybuilding instead of his law enforcement career, he would have been one of the best in the world. His knowledge of contest preparation is really second to none, having learned from the best after all. More importantly, Richard is brutally honest. If you don't look good, he will not tiptoe around it. He will be blunt.

Most bodybuilders can't handle that type of honesty, especially in today's age of social media. We have become accustomed to posting pics of ourselves online and having everyone blow sunshine up our butts. While that might feel good, it's not going to help you to be at your best. Quite the opposite. It is human nature to take our foot off the gas pedal if we feel we are ready. Why suffer anymore with low carbs? I look good. I don't need an extra cardio session. Everyone says I look great. What I knew I needed was honesty, along with knowledge.

It wasn't that I didn't know how to prepare. Every great athlete needs a good coach. Even Ali had Angelo Dundee in his corner. I had Richard. If I wasn't at my best, he would tell me. He would help me design a plan that would get me into my best possible shape. I was honoured that he agreed to help me prepare.

The first hurdle was time. The day I received my invite was exactly twelve weeks out from the contest. That is NOT a lot of time. I had been training, of course. It's part of my lifestyle as much as brushing one's teeth would be. Of course, there is training and eating healthy, and then there is contest prep training and eating—two very different animals.

Richard put together a very strict diet for me that had to start immediately. The training regimen was severe as well. I was introduced to giant sets, drop sets, supersets, and extreme intensity training. I would learn more in these twelve weeks than in the previous twelve years. God bless Gruskin and Richard Politano. I had a long way to go and not much time to get there.

The gym rallied around me. Members donated money to help with the expense of the whole adventure. My clients stepped up and bought training packages. All of my energy went towards training as hard as humanly possible. Train, eat, rest, train some more. Local news agencies picked up the story, and I found myself being interviewed on TV and radio. It wasn't just that I was invited to compete at the Mr. Universe that they were interested in. It was my journey from prison to the Universe that was of interest. My story was affecting people in a positive manner. This time, things were different.

When I was a kid, I dreamt of strength and muscle. Muscle as my personal armour. If I was big and strong, nobody could hurt me. I would maybe get the girl. It was my personal protection against becoming my father. I fell in love with the artistry of bodybuilding. It spoke to me on many levels. However, over time it became twisted. It became an ugly gargoyle of a thing. It became beyond selfish. My fears, insecurities, the demons from my past pain took over, or should I say, I let them take over. I wanted a pro card, money, anything to make the pain stop. I had to hit bottom. Had to.

Once at the bottom, I had that decision to make. Roll over and die or fight. Fighting meant being accountable. The hardest thing one must do in order to grow is to be accountable. Everyone has pain. Everyone has to go through challenges in life—some more than others. Pain is a part of life as much as pain is a part of training. You must suffer to grow. The most valuable lesson that I learned through this all was very simple, and if it helps anyone, then it was worth it.

That lesson is this: yes, some terrible things happened to me.

However, once I accepted responsibility for my actions, once I became accountable, everything changed for me. Yes, this was hard. It is hard to face your mistakes in life and look in the mirror and say, "Yup, that was my fault. That was a horrible decision. I need to be better than that!"

I blamed everything and everybody for my mistakes for a long time, until rock bottom. Another benefit to owning your actions is that they can't be used against you. That is an incredibly emancipating thing. Own it. You take away people's ability to weaponize your past against you.

This time, things were different. No longer was I concerned with glory or winning a pro card or making money or anything else that really did not mean much. This became an all-out war with my past, my mistakes, and my personal demons.

This contest became my chance to show other people that have faced tough obstacles in life that it is possible to turn things around to fulfill their dreams and goals. That it is possible to succeed in the face of adversity. I used everything as motivation. Everyone that would laugh at me when I started training with weights as a skinny teen. The anger towards my father. I thought of my Mother's sacrifices and hard work when I didn't want to train anymore. I thought of representing my country on a world stage. I walked up and down hills until my feet literally bled in the cold and rain at times.

All the while channeling the anger that I had towards myself for hurting good people in my life and the mistakes I made. This contest became my Apollo Creed—my title shot. Just like Rocky, I did not care if I won. I wanted to go the distance. To me, that meant emptying the tank completely. It did not matter to me if I came in dead last. Just by competing, I would be fulfilling the promise I made to an 18-year-old me so many years ago. I was going to do it or die trying.

I would remember that battered 13-year-old screaming out, "I'm not a loser!" after my first boxing match. I took all the pain, hurt, anger, and joy, and I used all of it. I would train and remember the last time I saw my father, remember the sick feeling in my gut when they told me died.

Tears would stream down my face as I trained beyond the pain, remembering trying to wake my Dad up in the garage. If nothing else, I would know that I mattered. It was not based on how I placed in the contest. This was an inner battle against everything I had allowed to hold me back. I would face my inner demons head-on and crush them once and for all! This was a different contest. This contest was, in my mind at least, a battle for everyone that had fallen down and dared to get back up.

"Life ain't all sunshine and rainbows."

Before I knew it, the longest and shortest twelve weeks of my life had passed by. I was going to England to compete, just like Arnold had—at the Mr. Universe competition!

My friend and client, Ralph Eannance, had flown all the way from New York to support me. Ralph is a New York State Judge. He had become a huge supporter and mentor to me during my darkest times while living in Saskatchewan. It was great having him there, a friendly face in the crowd. Whenever I was down, Ralph was there to listen and advise.

Before I ever reached the stage, I thought about all the people that had helped me. The Kliewer family and most notably my friend and brother Rob Kliewer. My basketball coaches, Syd Korsunsky and Ken Kelsh. Jimmy "Babyface" Saunders. Aubrey who believed in me when nobody else would give me a chance. My childhood friend Trevor King who showed endless patience with me as we grew up together. Everyone from King's Fitness that supported and helped me get to England in the first place.

The person I thought about the most was my Mom, Lucille, the toughest person I have ever known. Anything that is good in me came from her. If nothing else, I wanted to honour her. She was the hero. She fought the fight. I knew a bodybuilding contest would not mean much to her. I wanted to honour her in my effort, nevertheless—in my heart.

Birmingham, England. Here I was. About to walk in to register for the Mr. Universe contest. The room was packed. Past bodybuilding legends, coaches, press, executive, judges and of course competitors from all over the world. Large teams from the Eastern Bloc, Brazil, the UK, France, Italy. It was overwhelming. And then there was me in my CANADA hoodie I bought from the Bay. I talked to as many people as I could. I knew that this could very well be a once-in-a-lifetime experience, and I wanted to soak it all in.

I proceeded to make my way through the registration line and was greeted very warmly by Val Charles and her husband, Jim. Val made me feel at home immediately. I felt some of my tension evaporate. So far, England had been amazing.

A few days earlier, I had trained at Dorian Yates' (6-time Mr. Olympia winner) world-famous Temple Gym. While there, I ran into Ernie Taylor, retired Olympia competitor and bodybuilding royalty. He was amazing. After my workout, he put me through some posing and gave me many helpful pointers. I nervously asked him his opinion of my physique.

His words lifted me, "Mate, you look fantastic! Don't change a thing!"

My confidence rose a little bit. Maybe, just maybe, this would go all right!

The day had arrived. At the venue, the competitors were all relaxing, waiting for their class to be given the go-ahead to start pumping up before heading onstage. I spotted Mark Anderson from New Zealand. Mark was a previous Mr. Universe winner, and we had become friendly online in the weeks leading up to the show. I walked over to him, and he warmly greeted me. He invited me to sit down, and we spent the time chatting about all things bodybuilding. I had no idea how he looked under his tracksuit, although judging by his sunken face, it appeared he was in shape or, as they would say in the UK, "in good nick!"

Then the call came, "Masters Competitors, start warming up!" We all headed to the pump area to begin the process of pumping up for the stage. I felt a huge rush of adrenaline. Once in the pump-up area, everyone started to strip down to their posing trunks.

Any thoughts I may have had of winning quickly started to vanish as I saw the quality of physiques around. My first thoughts were, "Everyone looks fantastic!" It reminded me of how I felt at my first National competition. This was a different level. Not that the National level guys in Canada are not good, they are, very, in fact. But this…this was unreal. Pictures never do a physique justice. You have to see it in 3-D to truly get a sense of how someone looks.

I was shaken. Plain and simply shook to the core. I started to scan the room, looking for someone I thought I could beat. Over there, in the corner, was ONE guy from Greece, I think. Maybe, I could beat him.

Then Mark took off his tracksuit. The room became quieter. Mark looked crazy. It was as if someone had peeled his skin off. About ten days before I left for England, I had my body fat tested, and it registered at under 3% body fat. It was a skinfold test, so allowing for room for error, I was probably somewhere between 3-4% body fat. By the time of the show, possibly a touch leaner. I was shredded. By comparison, Mark looked like the world OWED him bodyfat. It did not look real.

It was pretty clear. Mark would win.

Then something happened within me. I smiled. I was happy for Mark. He looked incredible. He was a champion and a gentleman. True class. It would be an honour to share the stage with him. I would enjoy this! Screw it! I AM AT THE MR. UNIVERSE, AND I AM GOING TO ENJOY EVERY SECOND OF THIS!

"Number 107, step forward." Yes, they meant me. It hit me at that moment. I am doing it, really doing it, just like Arnold did. I stepped forward and felt my body begin to open up. The 18-year-old Todd smiled. Top six at the Mr. Universe. The skinny little kid from Elmwood. The kid that sometimes was afraid, the kid that took beatings from Jeffrey at Pan Am boxing club. The kid that was laughed at. The ex-con.

"Front double bicep, please, gentlemen."

BOOM! I hit the pose with confidence. Felt myself smiling despite myself. A few more poses were called. With each pose, I felt better, stronger.

"I AM REALLY HERE!"

I thought of my Mom. People were applauding as we went through our poses. It was electric.

"Rear double biceps, gentlemen."

I knew this was one of my stronger poses, and I hit it slowly and deliberately. I could hear people cheering as I hit the shot. They maneuvered us around the stage, and I was closer to the middle now, which is a good sign. I was being compared with the top guys. The pain, the exhaustion, it all fell away. I felt like I could pose forever.

And then, as quickly as it began, it was over.

It was now time to announce the placings and the winner. No matter what happened now, it didn't matter. I had done it. I had done what I had been told was impossible. From the inside of a jail cell to the most historic bodybuilding contest in the world. I had gone the distance. I emptied the tank and fought off all the pain, frustration, and every demon that had haunted me since that fateful day in the garage a lifetime ago.

"In fourth place, from Canada, TODD PAYETTE!"

FOURTH PLACE! Who would have thought? I was thrilled! They gave me a huge trophy and raised my hand. I think I was in shock, to be honest.

Mark did end up winning, deservedly so. It didn't matter. Fourth felt like first to me. I fought the good fight. I crushed the demons.

I will leave you with these thoughts...

It is ok to fail. It is not ok to quit. Be accountable. Own your mistakes and victories. There are enough people in this world that blame everyone and everything for their troubles. If you own it, you will grow and be stronger. You WILL succeed!

It's like Coach Korsunsky said to me so many years ago, "Shoulder Down."

Thank you, Coach.

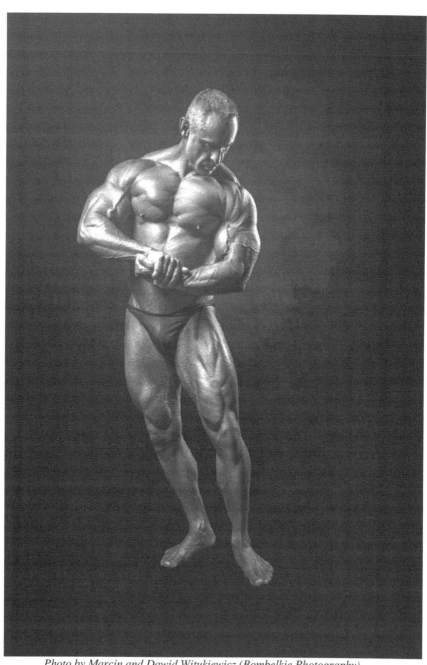

Photo by Marcin and Dawid Witukiewicz (Bombelkie Photography).

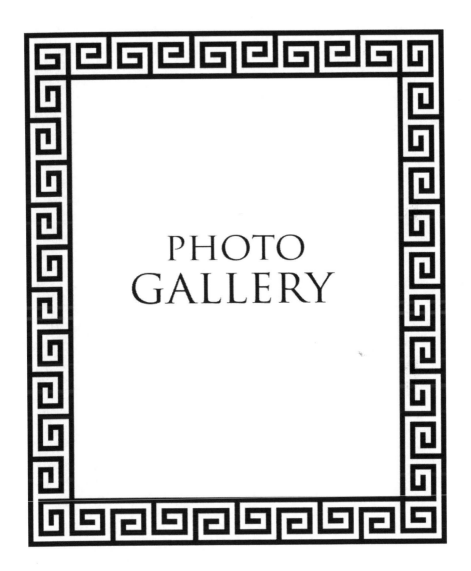

PHOTO
GALLERY

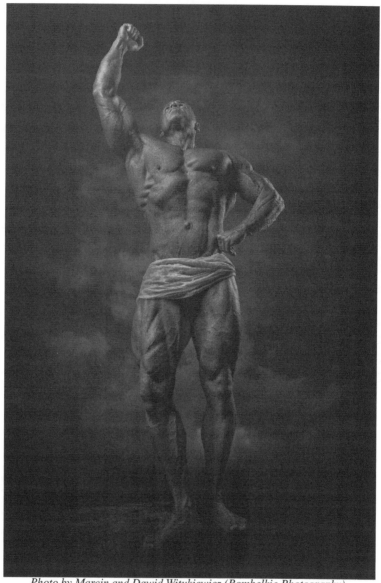

Photo by Marcin and Dawid Witukiewicz (Bombelkie Photography).

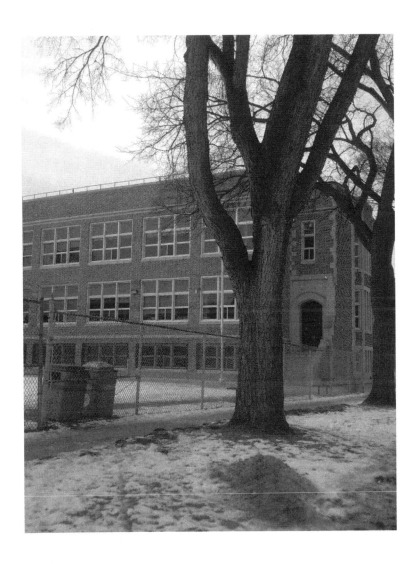

Glenelm School, where Mr. Neufeld patiently taught me how to hit a softball.
Trevor and I, as well as most of the kids in our little neighborhood, went there.
It was our home base.

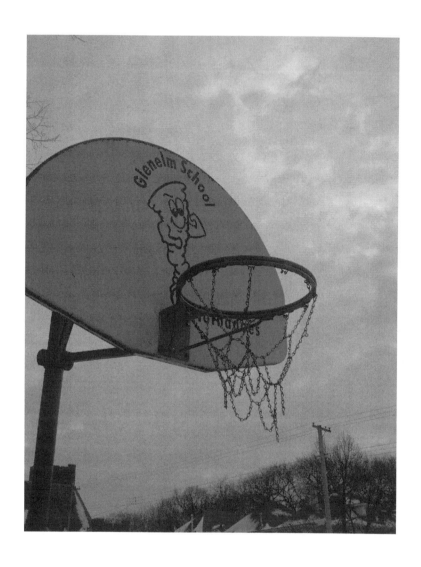

Countless hours were spent shooting at hoops just like this.

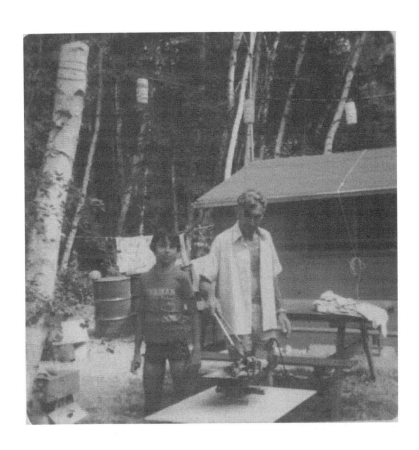

*Mr. Kliewer and I. "Bruno," Rob's father, was in many ways the closest thing
I had to one. This was at the Kliewer cottage. I was 11 years old. This was the
first day I ever ate a real steak!*

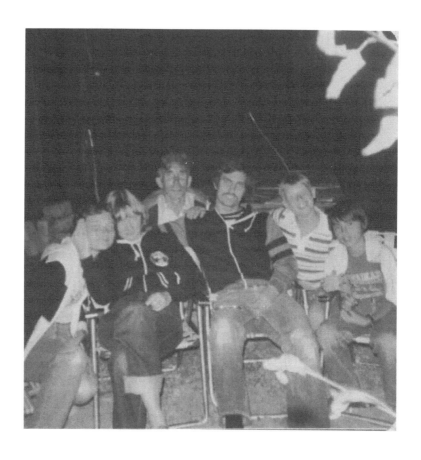

Almost the whole Kliewer family (Mrs. Kliewer took the pic).
L-R: Anita (Rob's sis), Faye (Rob's sister in law),Bruno (Dad), Vern (Rob's
brother), Rob and yours truly. I dearly love these folks.

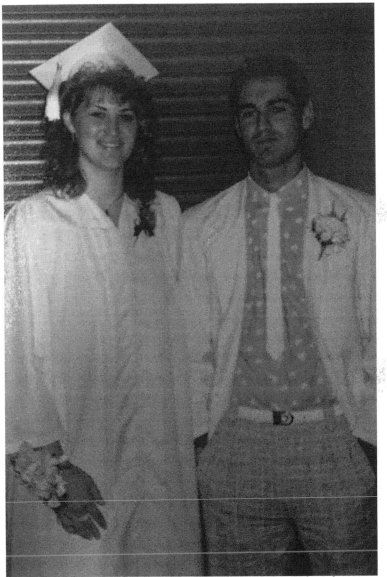

Now that's style!!! Gotta love the 80's. Taking the lovely Samantha to her prom.
She went with me, DESPITE my fashion sense! A great lady to this day.

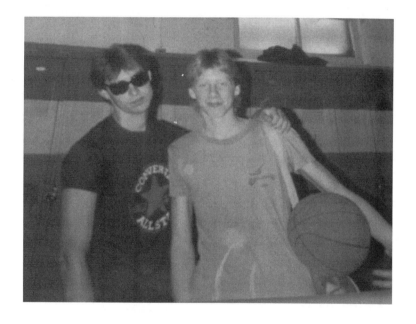

The 15 year old version. Certainly no evidence of a bodybuilding future in this pic. Trying my best to look very "Tom Cruise." Standing with my fellow basketball junkie, Mark Koop!

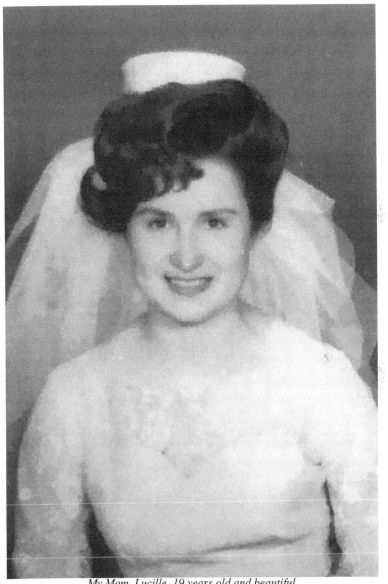

My Mom. Lucille. 19 years old and beautiful.
My favourite photo of her.

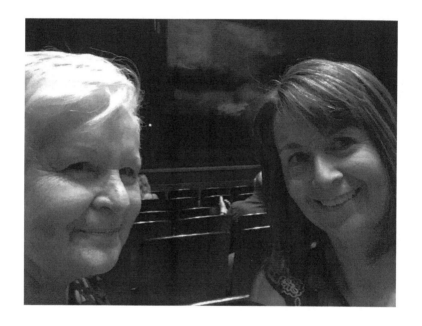

My Mom and big sis Linda. A night on the town.
Love them more than can be expressed.

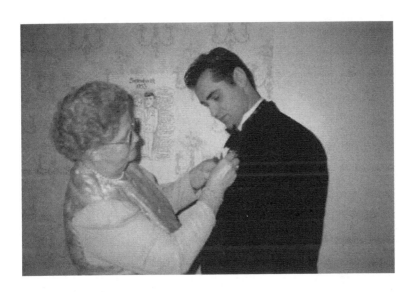

Mrs. Kliewer (Margaret) and myself on Rob's wedding day. She was the kindest woman I've ever met. I miss her terribly. She treated me as one of her own. So much love. Godspeed, Mrs. Kliewer.

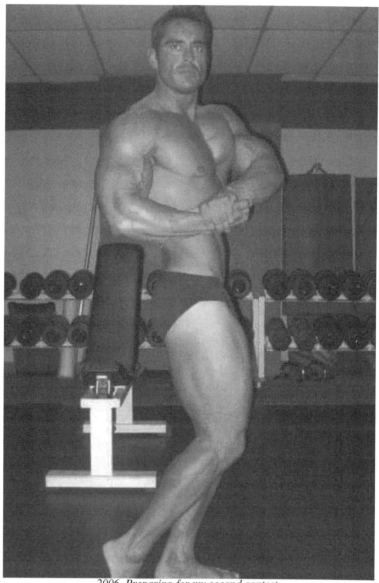

2006. Preparing for my second contest.
Can't believe I was that young.

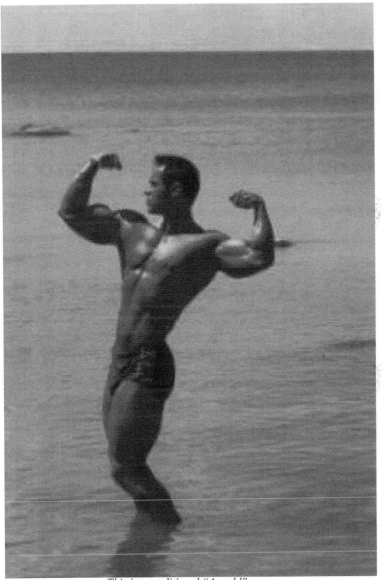

This is a traditional "Arnold" pose.
I stole, I mean, borrowed, many poses from him.

237

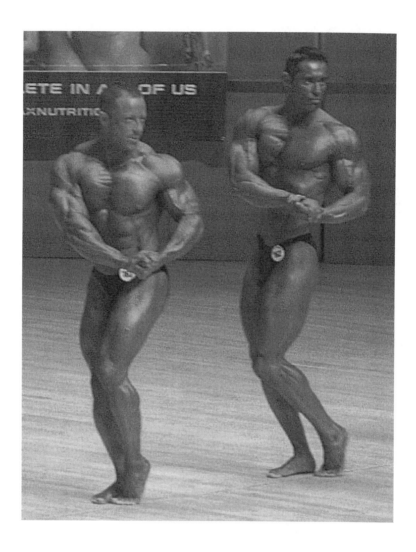

Onstage with fellow Winnipeg boy, Craig Bonnet. Competed against him three times, lost three times! He's a great champion, trainer and one of the funniest fellows around. 2007 Canadian Championships.

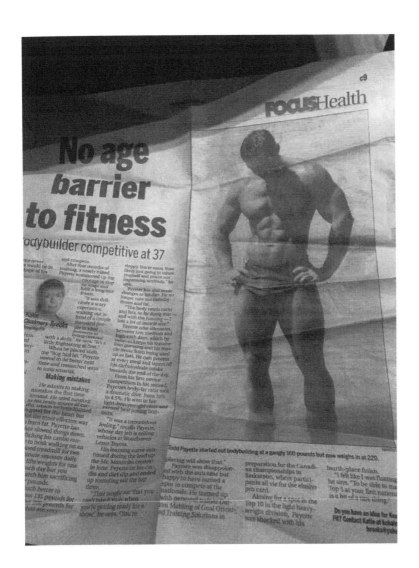

A little bit of local notoriety back in the day.

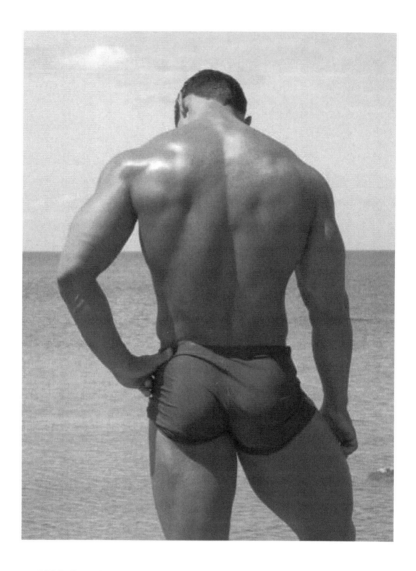

2006 Photo shoot. Another example of how a "non-posed" shot can look better than a posed one. I was literally trying to think of a pose to hit when the photographer snapped this.

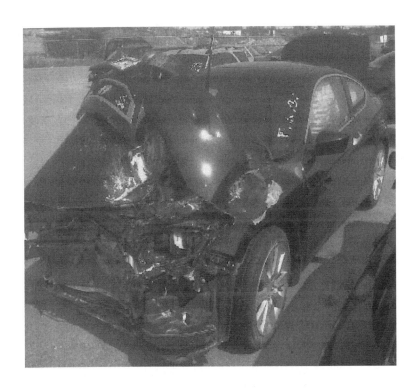

What was left of my car after the "accident."

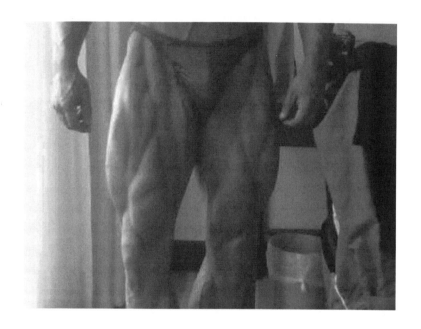

Checking out the legs at the hotel before the
2009 Canadian Bodybuilding Championships.

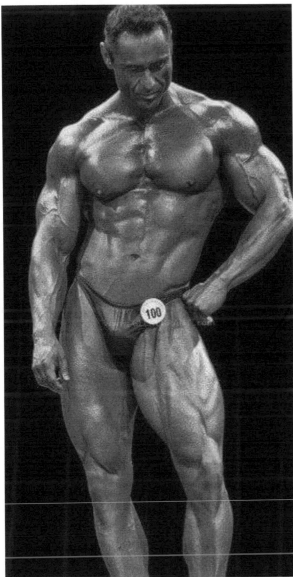

Sometimes the best pose is no pose at all. I envisioned the statue of David when I created this "non-pose". I would often begin my posing routines standing motionless in this stance as the music began to play. This photo, more than any other taken of me, represents my interpretation of the body as art.

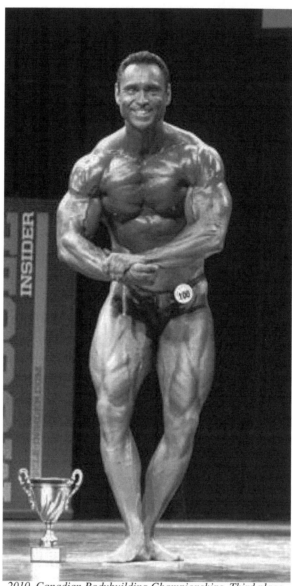

2010. Canadian Bodybuilding Championships. Third place.
One year before my life spiralled out of control.

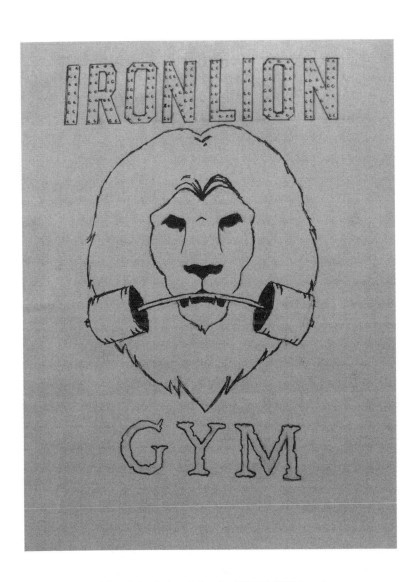

My original sketch for the IRONLION logo!

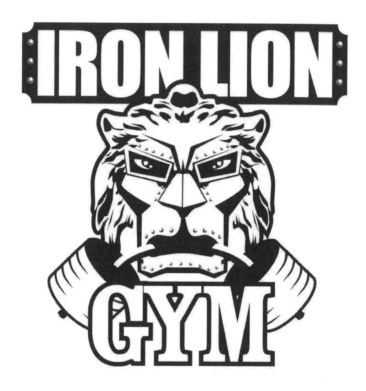

The first finished version.

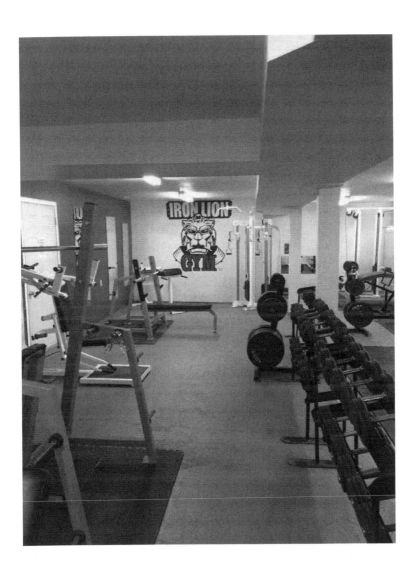

My little sanctuary. Miss this place.

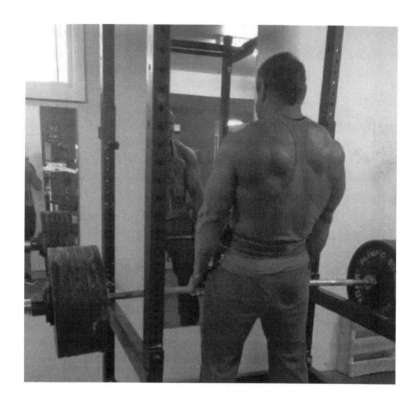

Sometimes you need to lift heavy things. Shrugs for trapezius development, about 600lbs on the bar.

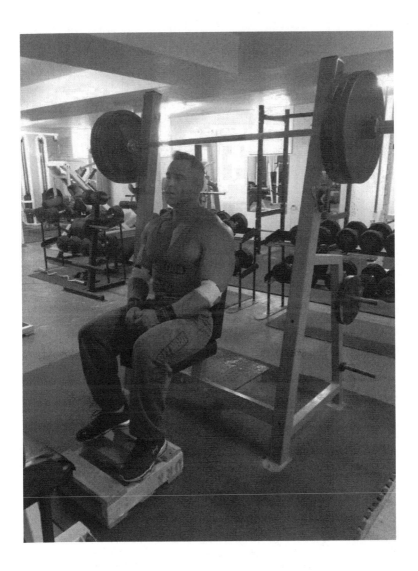

My face says it all. That's 315lbs on the bar. It has to be hoisted overhead. Time to get serious. FLIP THE SWITCH, BE THE MACHINE. Photo taken in IRONLION Gym.

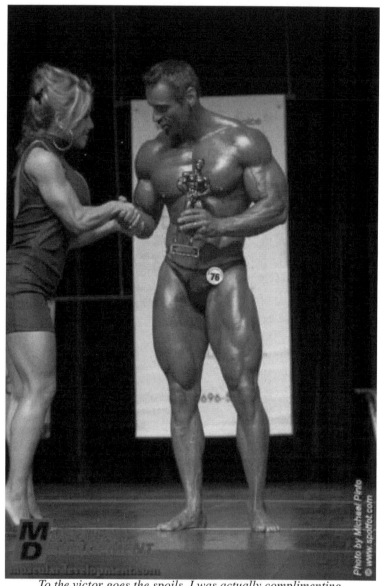

To the victor goes the spoils. I was actually complimenting
her on her dress despite what it looks like!

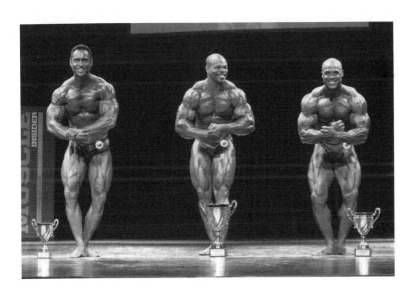

Top three at the 2010 Canadian Bodybuilding Championships.
1st Chris White, 2nd Tyrone Ashmeade, 3rd Todd something or other.

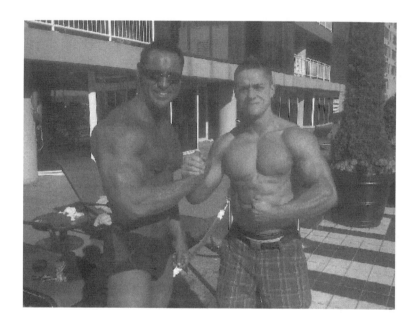

*Toronto. The day after the Canadian Bodybuilding Championships. Poolside
with fellow Winnipeger and National Junior Champion, Patric Gregoire.
My cookies and milk arrived 5 minutes after this photo was taken.*

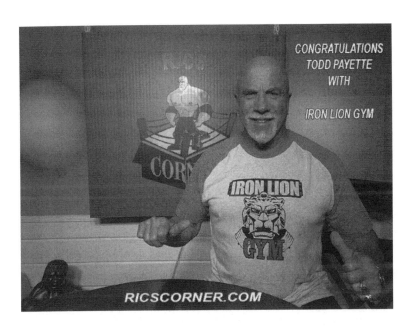

Bodybuilding legend and former training partner of Arnold Schwarzenegger himself. Ric Drasin! Ric designed the world famous logo's for both Golds Gym and Worlds Gym. He loved the IRONLION logo so much that I sent him a t-shirt. To my surprise, he wore it on his very popular YouTube show. Godspeed and Godbless you my brother in iron. RIP Ric.

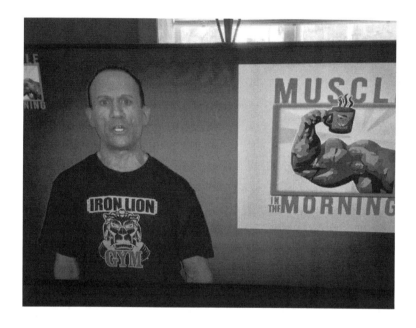

Dave Palumbo. Bodybuilding guru, owner of Species Nutrition and host of the extremely popular RX MUSCLE bodybuilding show, repping my IRONLION t-shirt. Dave's show is the number one go to for all things fitness. His knowledge of bodybuilding training and preparation is among the world's best!!!

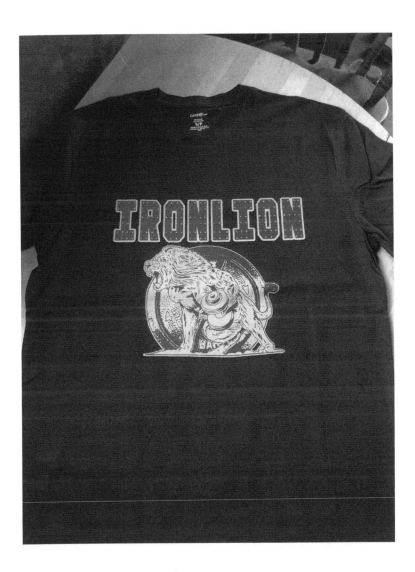

The current IRONLION logo was designed by Jeff Preston.
Jeff is a world renowned illustrator and also an avid weight trainer
and a fan of bodybuilding!

255

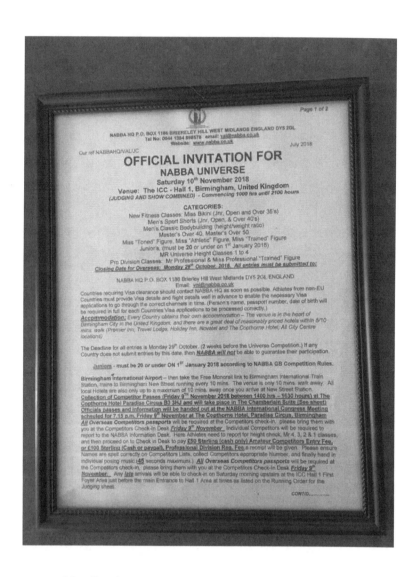

My official NABBA Universe invite framed for posterity.

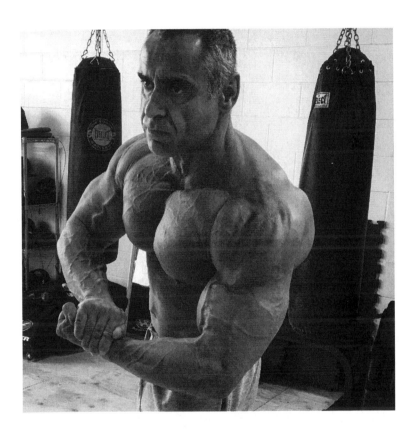

Posing, posing and more posing! Truly an art form, and is much harder than it looks. Getting ready for the Universe!

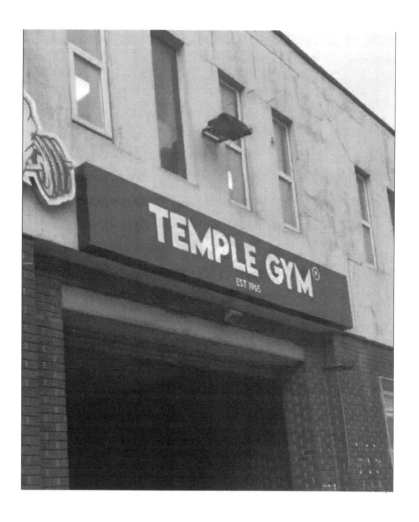

*Birmingham, England. The legendary and champion producing
"Temple Gym." It was a great experience to be able to walk through
those doors and train.*

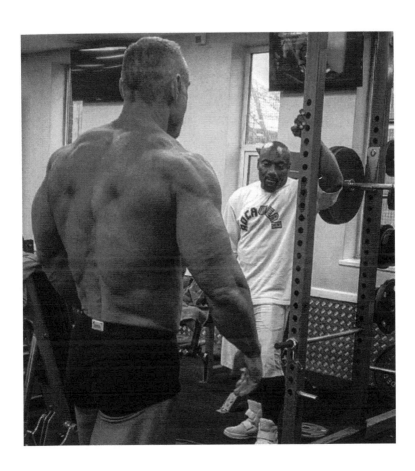

The great Ernie Taylor, former Mr. Olympia contender, putting me
through my paces the week before the Mr. Universe.
A great guy, legend!

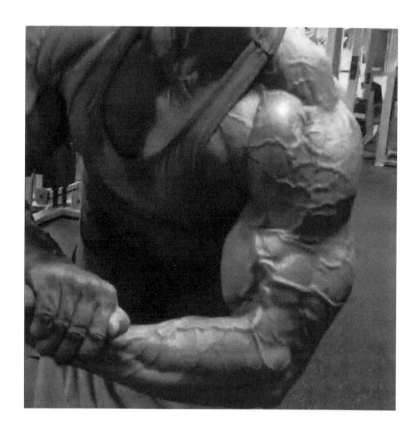

Two weeks before the Universe. The sharpest conditioning I have ever achieved. You truly have to suffer to get this low in bodyfat.

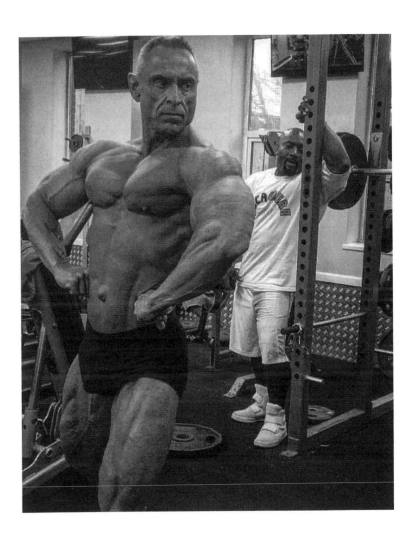

Never posed harder in the gym than this day. Ernie Taylor is a true posing master! Temple Gym.

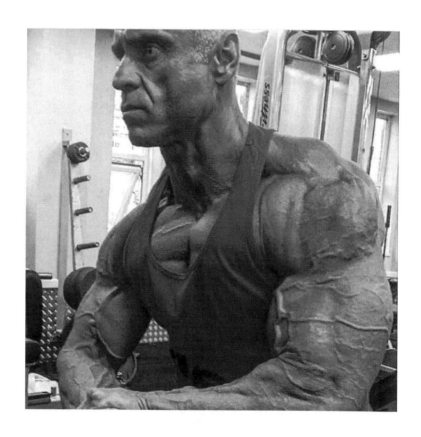

*Training at Dorian Yates world famous "Temple Gym"
in Birmingham, England.*

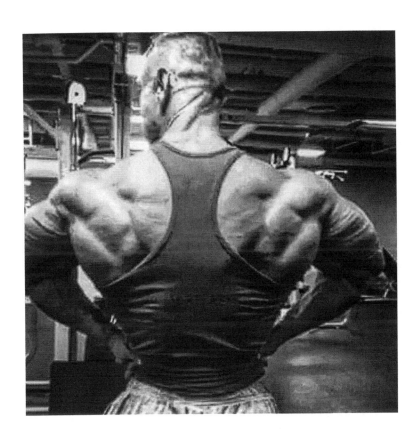

The old adage is "bodybuilding shows are won from the back!"

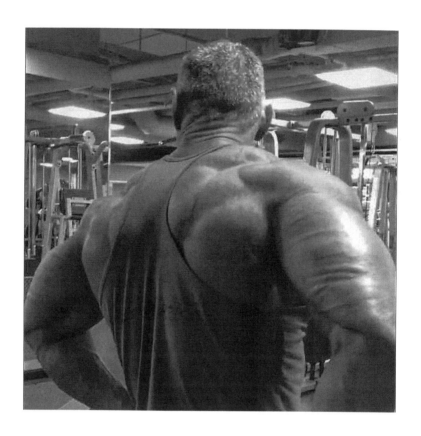

A couple weeks out from the Universe and trying to decide on the next exercise. All while dreaming of donuts!

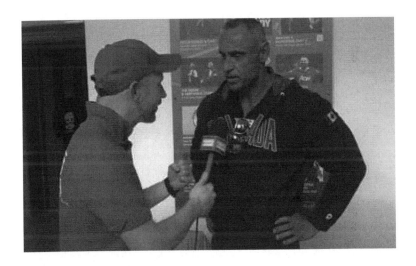

Being interviewed by Kris Clarke of "Pumped Media."
He loved my "Arnold" impression. Kris is a class act.

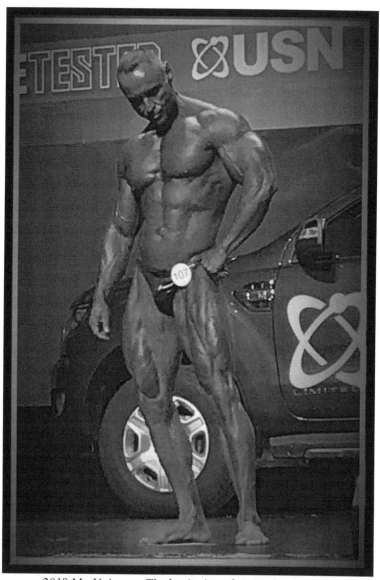

2018 Mr. Universe. The beginning of my posing routine.
Hoping to God I don't forget what poses to hit!

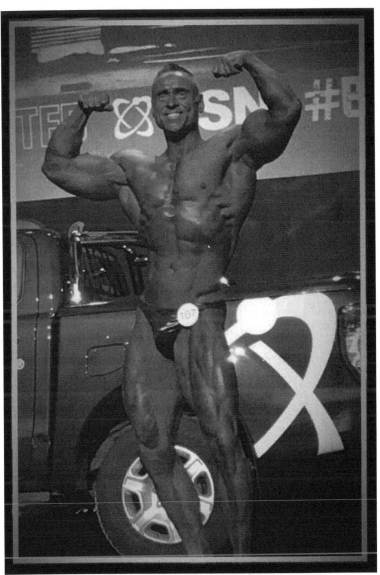

I just kept on smiling and hoping!

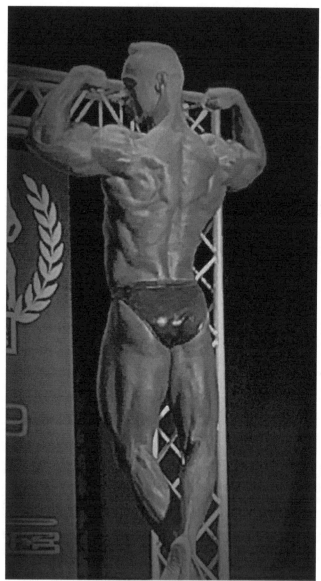

Mr. Universe. One of my fave poses.

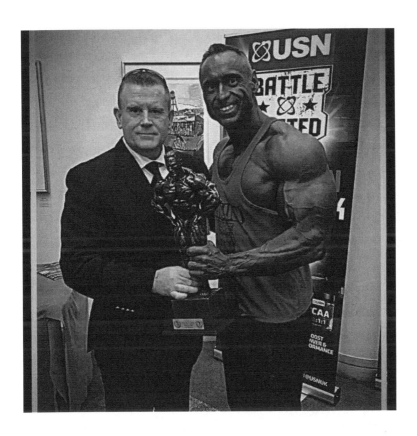

Yup, I'm tired, depleted, hungry. But look at that smile. Standing with a true gentleman of bodybuilding, NABBA's Si Sweeney. That 4th place trophy would never have happened without Si! "Onwards and upwards" as he always says!!! Love him like a brother.

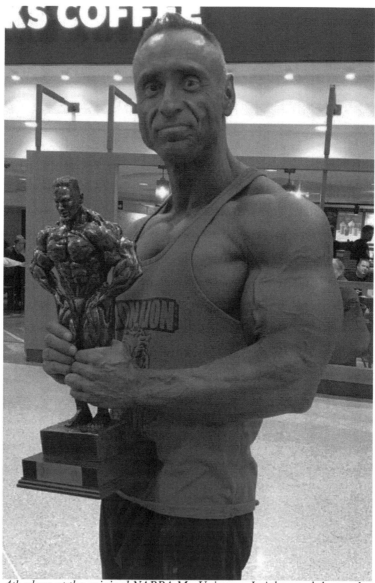

4th place at the original NABBA Mr. Universe. I nicknamed the trophy "Henri" after big Henry. "Don't feel bad if you're last!" Thanks Henry. Godspeed and RIP my iron brother.

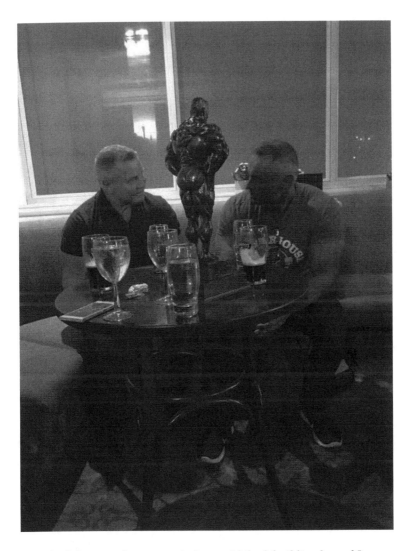

I had the great fortune to sit down with bodybuilding legend Ian Lawrence after the Mr. Universe competition. He has competed against the best ever in the bodybuilding world, including Arnold himself. It was a thrill to listen to his stories as "Henri" watched over the proceedings.

271

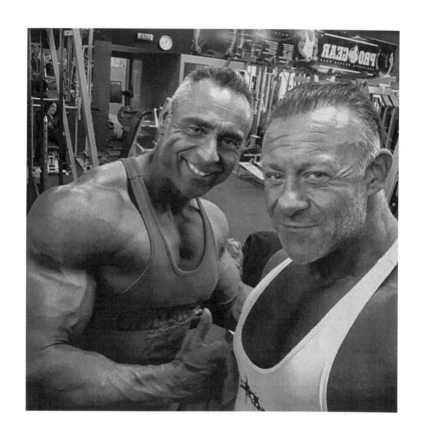

With Mr. Universe, Andy James. It was an honour to share the stage with him. I also had the privilege to hit a few incredible workouts with him! He's an animal!

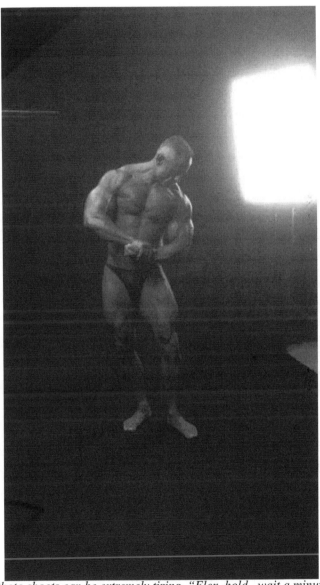

Photo shoots can be extremely tiring. "Flex, hold...wait a minute.
Light adjustment. Flex again...hold!" Captured for posterity!

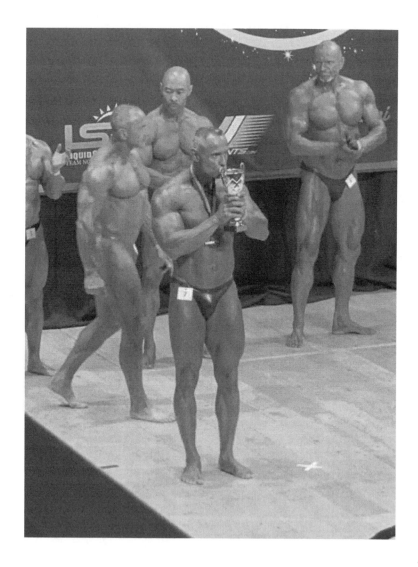

A fifth place finish at NABBA World Championships in Ireland. 2019.

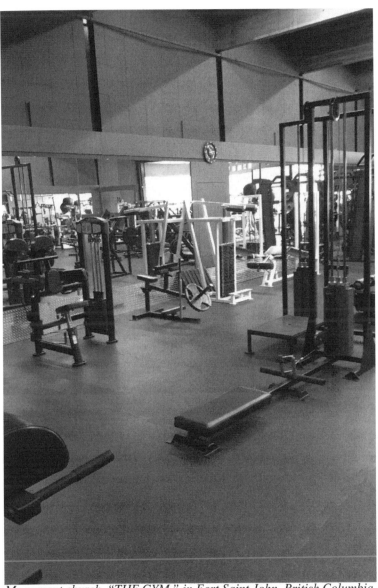

My current church, "THE GYM," in Fort Saint John, British Columbia.
Owned by the great IFBB pro, Jeni Briscoe.

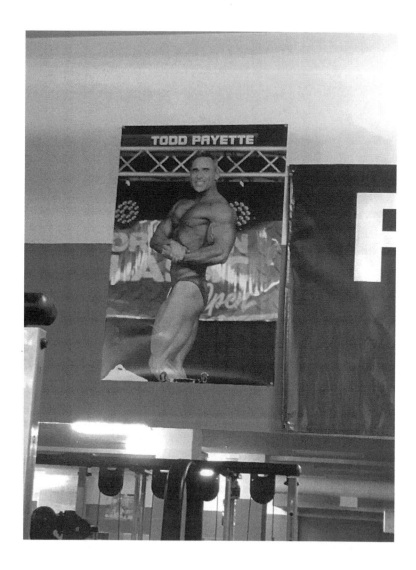

Look! I'm officially a big deal! Ok, so not really. Still humbled that
True North Fitness Centre hung a poster of me in their gym!
If you are ever in Dawson Creek, British Columbia, drop in.
It's an awesome training facility!

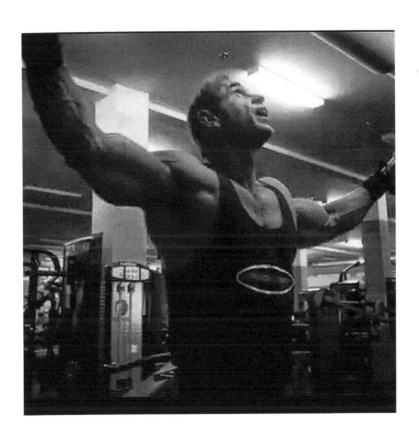

Training in 2021. The gym is still my safe haven.

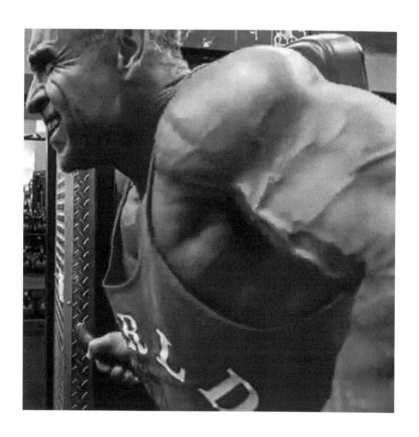

Still training hard at 52 years of age. Old dog, can't learn new tricks?
Or something like that! Can't remember the quote exactly.
Senility is not kind!

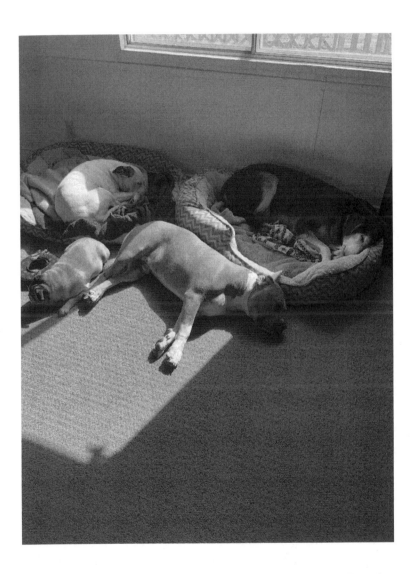

My kids. From left to right, Pugsley, Bella, Apollo and the old gentle soul...Rocco. These four are a true gift from God.

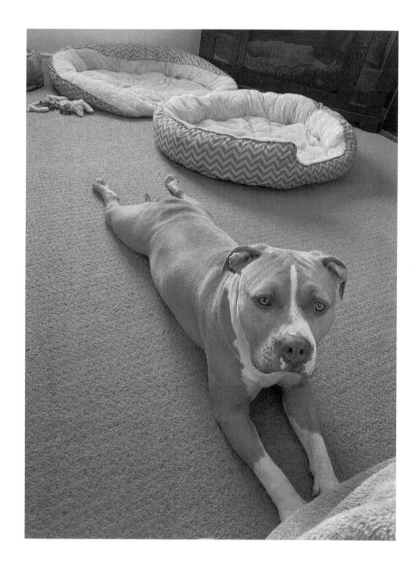

"Don't hate me because I'm beautiful!"
Apollo being...well, Apollo!

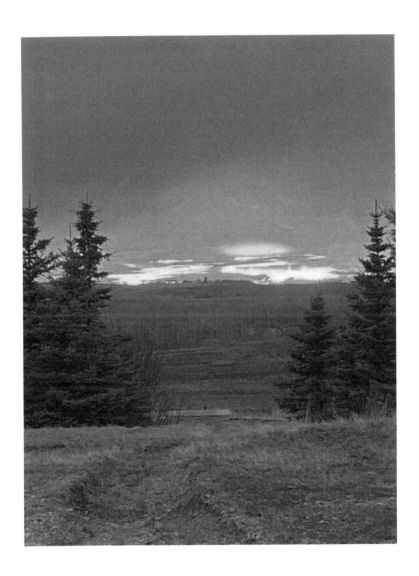

Where I live now. I found peace.
There is no greater thing.

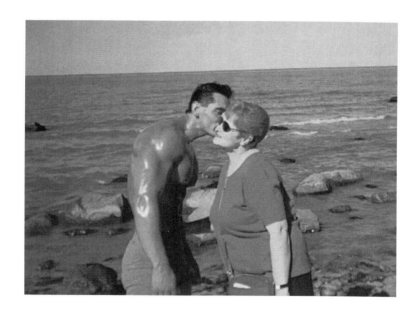

My Mom and I at one of my favourite spots, Victoria Beach, Manitoba.
Well before all the bodybuilding craziness!

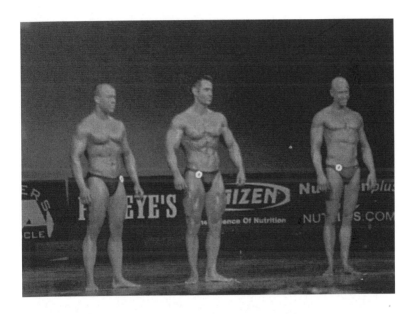

My second time around in the Manitoba Novice Bodybuilding Championships.
The true beginning of my strange odyssey in the world of all things muscle!

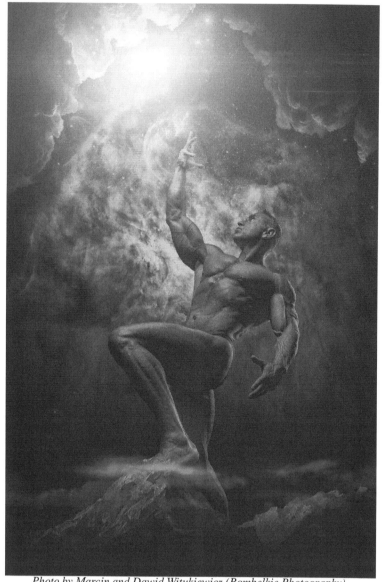

Photo by Marcin and Dawid Witukiewicz (Bombelkie Photography).

Made in the USA
Middletown, DE
14 July 2021